The Medicine Today Series
General Editor: DR CECIL HELMAN

Also in The Medicine Today Series

HYPNOSIS
a guide for patients and practitioners
by DAVID WAXMAN

ACUPUNCTURE

from Ancient Art to Modern Medicine

by

ALEXANDER MACDONALD

MB, BS, DLO

London
GEORGE ALLEN & UNWIN
Boston   Sydney

**George Allen & Unwin (Publishers) Ltd,
40 Museum Street, London WC1A 1LU, UK**

George Allen & Unwin (Publishers) Ltd,
Park Lane, Hemel Hempstead, Herts HP2 4TE, UK

Allen & Unwin Inc.,
9 Winchester Terrace, Winchester, Mass 01890, USA

George Allen & Unwin Australia Pty Ltd,
8 Napier Street, North Sydney, NSW 2060, Australia

First published 1982

British Library Cataloguing in Publication Data

Macdonald, Alexander
Acupuncture: from ancient art to modern
medicine. – (Medicine today series)
1. Acupuncture
I. Title   II. Series
615.8'92   RM184
ISBN 0-04-616023-X

Set in 11 on 12 point Bembo by Nene Phototypesetters Ltd
and printed in Great Britain by
Mackays of Chatham

Acknowledgements

◆

I am indebted to my wife's understanding and enthusiastic support. I would like to thank my patients for providing invaluable information I required to develop my ideas about acupuncture. I would also like to give my warmest appreciation to all my colleagues who have freely given me so many ideas: particularly Dr Felix Mann, who first introduced me to the subject and encouraged me to continue my work; Roger Greenhalgh, Professor Harding Rains, Dr Bacha Master and Dr Tony Rubin, who have given me the facilities to investigate the subject using Western medical methods; Drs Lu Gwei-Djen and Joseph Needham, who have not only given me their inspiration but have also provided the invaluable material in their book *Celestial Lancets*; Dr John Lin Chung Zhi, who has provided me with a wealth of information about the Chinese medical practice; and Dr Peter Nathan, who directed my first footsteps in attacking the mountains of scientific papers that are relevant to a modern understanding of acupuncture. I am also extremely grateful to Dr Ilza Veith and the University of California Press for their generosity in allowing me to quote so extensively from her translation of *The Yellow Emperor's Classic of Internal Medicine*.

I should also like to thank Dr Cecil Helman, general editor of the Medicine Today Series; my publishers and Peter Leek in particular, for their patient yet persuasive direction of my early drafts; and Michael Radford for his careful attention to detail. In addition, I would like to thank Stewart Ganley for his line illustrations. A number of these were based on published or traditional sources with some adaptation or modification. I am indebted to the following:

Figure 9   Documenta Geigy, *Scientific Tables*, 6th Ed.

Figure 12   Felix Mann, *The Meridians of Acupuncture* (Heinemann Medical Books Ltd, 1972) pp. 143–146.

Figure 13   George Soulié de Morant, *L'Acuponcture Chinoise, Atlas* (Maloine S.A. Éditeur-Paris, 1972) fig. 69.

Figures 14, 17 and 18   Felix Mann, *Acupuncture, The Ancient Chinese Art of Healing* (Heinemann Medical Books Ltd, 1978) fig. 62, p. 153; fig. 37, p. 88; and fig. 38, p. 89.

Figure 19   William Lowe, *Introduction to Acupuncture Anesthesia* (Medical Examination Publishing Company, 1973) fig. 11, p. 82.

Thanks are also due to the Wellcome Trustees for permission to reproduce Plates 1, 2, 3 and 7; and to WHO for the photos that make up Plates 5 and 6 by D. Henrioud.

Finally, my tireless secretaries, both named Cynthia, without whose dedicated work none of this would have been possible, will be pleased indeed to see their manuscript translated into book form.

Contents

◆

painless treatment – Moxibustion – The difference between
acupuncture and moxibustion

PART THREE MODERN ACUPUNCTURE

List of illustrations

◆

Introduction

◆

Three vital questions:
How on earth do the needles work?
How successful is acupuncture for my type of complaint?
How painful is the treatment?

If ever you wish to seek the aid of acupuncture for the first time, ask the practitioner these questions. I hope this book will arm you with enough information to assess his replies during the first consultation and discover for yourself what sort of doctor he is, and how he intends to treat you.

I have divided the book into three parts, which need not necessarily be read in sequence. The first is but a brief chapter describing the clash between traditional and modern medicine in China; the second summarises the relevant aspects of traditional Chinese medicine; while the third introduces the reader to modern Western developments.

How do the needles work?
Patients sitting in the waiting-room before meeting an acupuncturist for the first time must often wonder if they have come to the right place at all. Desperation alone drives most patients to his doors, particularly when conventional Western medical methods have failed to provide sufficient relief from their illness. Will such an 'unorthodox' form of treatment be the answer? How can it possibly work, when the Western 'scientific' approach has failed?

These hopes and fears are the natural feeding-ground for any practitioner who wishes to exploit the apparently non-sensical and almost mystical aspects of the subject described in Part Two of this book.

Modern Western medical methods are little more than two
and a half centuries old. When a patient has not responded to
them, it is easy to suggest that the Chinese have developed
their ideas over the past two and a half millennia and, therefore,
have discovered something that we in the West are not mature
enough to understand. Indeed, blinkered by science Western
medicine may appear to the discontented patient to have
galloped off in entirely the wrong direction.

This book hopes to show that this story is just not true.
Medical thinking in China was similar to that found in many
other systems of medicine developed in the ancient civilis-
ations of Egypt, Greece, India, Islam, Mesopotamia and
Rome.

In those days physicians who had the intellectual capacity to
stand back and reflect on the causes of disease without the aid
of microscopes, X-rays and all the modern technical developments of medicine were all driven to similar conclusions. Why
did these ideas persist for so long in China, when in the West
they have been eclipsed by the dramatic achievements of
modern medicine? The simplest explanation, put forward in
Chapter 1, is that the Chinese themselves did not become
involved in modern medical methods until the twentieth
century. Every medical student today in China has to learn
anatomy, for example: until the 1920s this vital part of a
modern doctor's understanding of medicine was not possible
in China; thitherto everyone had a duty to return their bodies
intact to their ancestors.

Although it is easy enough to see something, one's inner
perception and understanding are sharpened and altered by
experience. Doctors from the traditional and Western schools
of medicine in present-day China perceive the causes of
disease in different ways according to their training. However, the Chinese may be building a bridge between the two
schools at this moment. Many of the old ideas that sustained
the practice of acupuncture, for example, may be modified in
the future to allow the subject to rest more securely in a
modern mould; meanwhile Western medicine, as we will see
in Part Three of the book, has not been slow to criticise
several incorrect though highly cherished notions of the past.

I spoke recently to an experienced Chinese surgeon, who

told me that one of his duties was to teach the 'barefoot doctors' acupuncture. I wondered if he taught them the traditional approach that will be described in Part Two of this book. He smiled and said that he could not possibly teach a system that he did not understand himself. He taught the barefoot doctors to insert needles in such and such a place for such and such a condition described in a straightforward Western manner.

I asked him how long it would take him to begin to use the traditional system of medicine developed in his own country; he told me that he would require three years of full-time apprenticeship to one of the well-known masters of the subject.

I then asked him how long it would take me, a Western-trained doctor, to learn to practise traditional acupuncture. He felt that once I had mastered the language and learnt to read Classical Chinese it would probably take me five years' work in China to achieve the necessary understanding of an approach so different from my own.

How successful is acupuncture for my type of complaint?

How can a Western-trained doctor practise such a subject successfully without knowing the language and spending five years in China? The answer is that we have the privilege of adopting only those parts of the system that appear to make sense in the light of our own understanding of medicine; for instance, I would hope that no Western doctor would use acupuncture as his first line of treatment in diabetes or an acute surgical emergency in the abdomen. Yet not so long ago traditional Chinese medicine was the only method available to patients living in China.

We in the West can afford to learn from Chinese experience in treating those conditions that are not easily treated in other ways. The best example of this is chronic pain. Here the Chinese have described in a remarkable wealth of detail many phenomena associated with chronic pain. As we will see, the similarities between Western and Chinese observations in this field are too great to ignore.

We now know that inserting a needle has a profound effect

on the nervous system. The nervous system's role in maintaining such conditions as chronic pain is so complex that it will never be fully understood. Nevertheless, we have evidence that the insertion of a needle may produce sufficient effects to break the vicious circle within the nervous system and on occasion produce sustained relief.

Acupuncture may help other illnesses where the nervous system has an important part to play. Nasal conditions such as sinusitis and hay fever may be included. Asthma and eczema, for example, may be partially relieved for long periods of time.

The symptoms of diseases such as cancer or tuberculosis may be relieved to some extent by acupuncture; but the diseases themselves are not altered by the treatment. In fact the dangers of masking such serious conditions will be mentioned again in Part Three of this book.

How painful is the treatment?
Does it hurt? The best way of answering this important question is to ask the acupuncturist to demonstrate the technique on himself. The confidence he displays when he inserts a needle into himself will tell you a great deal. The patient and practitioner should come to terms with each other to produce the most effective method of relief with the minimum amount of needling.

The acupuncturist is like the fisherman who wants to make the biggest catch with the finest line placed in exactly the right spot. Only his skill and experience will tell him how much to give each patient and where to insert the needle. A patient who has been in poor health and has already been fully investigated and treated in the appropriate Western manner will have few qualms about the insertion of needles that are much finer than injection needles. Provided the needling is carried out skilfully, there is little danger and, in appropriate circumstances, a great deal of relief is given, often within minutes.

Many patients start off with the idea that enormously long needles are used in acupuncture; perhaps they have seen them on television being used for a major operation. This aspect of acupuncture is described in Chapter 12 and received a great deal of publicity in the 1970s. However, it forms only a small part of the practice of acupuncture. Chronic conditions usually require shorter needles inserted to a depth of an inch or so. Indeed, some practitioners perform their work by inserting needles quite painlessly into the skin (see Figure 1).

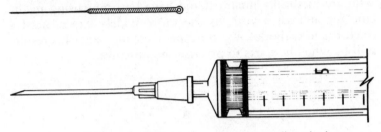

Figure 1   *Compare the thickness of an acupuncture needle with a hypodermic needle used in Western medicine.*

Where can I find a suitably qualified practitioner?
The first problem is to decide which sort of acupuncture you wish to have. If you believe that traditional Chinese acupuncture is required, you must find a practitioner who has been taught to read classical Chinese and has spent a number of years studying with the great masters of the subject in China. There are few practitioners of this type in the West.

If, on the other hand, you would prefer a more modern approach accompanied by a medical opinion, then you must make sure that your practitioner is on the medical register.

This will ensure that you will receive treatment when it is appropriate; in other words, the doctor will naturally avoid masking symptoms of diseases that should be treated in the conventional Western manner. Furthermore, he is likely to be conversant with many developments in the subject, which can only be practised by someone who is medically trained and has a special interest in your type of condition.

Those doctors who employ acupuncture for the relief of chronic pain, for example, will have taken a special interest in this part of medicine and have gained many ideas from Western-trained doctors who knew nothing about acupuncture. In the United Kingdom the best way to find such a practitioner is to ask your general practitioner's advice.

Doctors who wish to discover more about the subject
Doctors who wish to study the modern developments in
more detail are very welcome to write to me, as I hold short
courses with the aim of demonstrating the practical aspects of
the ideas found in Part Three of this book.

However, it is important to note that I only accept those
who are medically qualified and have been practising medicine for at least a year, as the more widely experienced a
doctor is in orthodox Western medicine the better his results
will be when he starts to practise acupuncture.

Part One

Ancient Art v. Modern Medicine

1
Swing of the Pendulum

—————◆—————

What are the effects of acupuncture? Can arthritis and other chronically painful conditions (such as backache and migraine) be cured or even helped by acupuncture? Are the effects of acupuncture 'all in the mind' as most lay and medical people outside China believe?

Even Joshua Horn, a British surgeon respected by the Chinese for the work he carried out in Peking since the Second World War, appeared to hold a similar opinion:

> The pelvic injury must have bruised the nerves to the bladder for the patient was unable to pass urine. To deal with this we called in a colleague from the acupuncture department. The Chinese traditional doctor, bearded and dignified, felt the pulse, nodded sagely and in a completely matter-of-fact way, told the patient that his problem would be solved immediately. This unbounded confidence in the efficacy of their treatment is characteristic of traditional doctors and probably contributes not a little to their success. He cleaned the skin with alcohol and iodine and, with a delicate twirling motion, inserted five acupuncture needles into the chosen spots. Within a few minutes the patient was able to pass urine and from that time onward he had no further bladder trouble.[1]

Whether the effective part of acupuncture is just suggestion and nothing more is a question which cannot be answered in one sentence; it will take the whole book to debate this.

Natural scepticism
Most Western doctors have been sceptical. A typical comment was made by a physician from Montpellier, journeying into China in 1767: 'Praise be to God not to have shown me one confirmation of the Chinese methods in my travels.' He was delighted not to have to re-think all he had learned in his medical school.

Most Western doctors today share his opinion. This is a natural reaction for anyone who has begun his studies in medical school by spending hundreds of hours dissecting cadavers, looking down microscopes at sections of tissues and performing experiments to unravel the internal mechanisms of the body. A Western medical student can state quite bluntly that never once during his arduous studies has he ever seen evidence of the 'meridians' described by traditional acupuncturists as an important arrangement of channels in the body.

Chinese anatomical studies
Some anatomical studies were performed in Ancient China, particularly on the battlefield: the lengths of the larger blood vessels were measured, and the circulation of the blood through organs of the body was described in China two thousand years before this idea was considered in Europe. Nevertheless, the anatomical studies carried out in Europe during the last four hundred years were not possible in China until the early 1920s; the Chinese believed that their bodies belonged to their ancestors and had to be returned to them intact. In addition, Confucian scholars tended to avoid soiling their hands in such odorous and practical activities as anatomy when they were able to pursue a more elegant path debating the many meanings of ancient medical manuscripts.

For the first time in the 1920s bodies of executed criminals were allowed to be dissected in the anatomy departments of the new medical schools pioneered by missionary societies in China. A professor of anatomy complained that the executions were so clumsy that his students could not study the neck region properly. The local warlord told him that if he persisted with his complaint the prisoners would be sent to his department and the professor could execute them in any way he wished.[2]

Despite these early difficulties, anatomy departments in China have been conducting their studies in a similar fashion to the West for the past fifty years. No Chinese scientist has ever reported any evidence of the existence of a discrete channel system that would explain the 'meridians'. Although in science it is impossible to prove something does *not* exist, it is possible to discount any faulty evidence or at least to state that no evidence to support a claim has been found.

So it is with some justification that a Western-trained doctor can tell his patient that he sees no reason why he should learn the principles of traditional acupuncture. When he has already mastered the essentials of the scientific approach to medicine and has had first-hand experience in applying these lessons in a very practical way for the benefit of his patients, it is a little hard to expect him to abandon all this in favour of an entirely different approach to diagnosis and treatment. For the concepts of traditional acupuncture share very little with those of scientific medicine.

Traditional medicine was at its lowest ebb in the early part of this century in China. Even its stoutest defenders would admit that it had fallen into the wrong hands; for there were large numbers of lower-grade doctors or apothecaries, itinerant medicine pedlars, and charlatans of every description. Dr William Sewell described his experiences when he first arrived in China during the 1920s to teach medical students chemistry. He saw an acupuncturist take a long needle out of one patient, wipe it on the side of his boot and polish it on his lapel before plunging it through layers of clothing into the next. What was perhaps more serious was the patients' habit of consulting one traditional doctor after another – to collect the herbal remedies each prescribed and consume them all simultaneously; the hospitals admitted many patients dying from herbal overdoses.[2]

Chinese attacks on traditional medicine
Some of the most serious attacks on traditional methods came from China herself during this century; for instance 60,000

people died in Manchuria of a plague between 1910 and 1911. Eighty traditional physicians were specially selected to control the plague. They all died of it themselves. The only person who was able to help was a young Cambridge-trained doctor, Wu Lien-te, who used his scientific knowledge to direct the sanitary and public health measures required to prevent the plague from spreading further. This made a great impression on the authorities. The venerable and hitherto traditionally oriented Viceroy of Manchuria, Hai Liang, remarked:

> The lessons taught us by this epidemic . . . have been great and have compelled several of us to revise our former ideas . . . if railways, telegraphs, electric lights, and other modern inventions are indispensable to the material welfare of this country, we should also make use of the wonderful resources of Western medicine for the benefit of our people.[3]

At the end of the First World War, the new generation of Chinese intellectuals were Western-oriented; they denounced many of their own traditions. Ch'en Tu-hsiu had harsh words to say about traditional medical beliefs:

> Our doctors don't know science. They don't understand human anatomy and what is more don't analyse the nature of medicine. As for bacteria and communicable diseases, they haven't heard of them. They only talk about the five elements, their production and elimination, heat and cold, *yin* and *yang*, and prescribe medicine according to old formulae. All these nonsensical ideas and reasonless beliefs must be cured by the support of science.[4]

Another intellectual, Lu Hsün, wrote short essays ridiculing traditional medical ideas, and succeeded in painting a horrifying picture of the superstitions that prevailed. In his story *Tomorrow*, he describes the traditional physician at work: 'He is ignorant and callous, brushing off the anxious queries of a widowed mother with empty phrases about "obstruction of the digestive tract" and "fire overpowering metal", in order to pocket his fee and be rid of her. After taking his prescription, the woman's son dies.'[5]

Traditional medicine's return to grace

Oil and wind up an old clock; its pendulum may continue to swing. Chinese patients continued to demand traditional acupuncture despite their leaders' criticisms; even some of the most ardent of modern physicians were forced to use traditional remedies for their own afflictions. Dr Hu Shih addressed doctors who had just qualified at his own University of Peiping: 'The old-style medicine will sooner or later be replaced by the modern.' However, when he himself developed diabetes before the days of insulin, he consulted a traditional doctor, Lu Chung-an, who completely cured him with herbs; not surprisingly, Dr Hu Shih was never able to condemn traditional medicine completely.[6]

Until recent times the only medicine known to most of China was traditional. In 1949, 95 per cent of Chinese doctors were of the traditional school. By the 1960s, however, less than half the Chinese doctors were traditional; their legacy of two millenia has persisted, and Chinese patients continue to demand traditional medicine. Recently an observer of a Canton rural commune noted that the proportions of patients requesting traditional as opposed to modern medicine were three to one.[7] It is probable that the Chinese belief in their traditional remedies has ensured that, for every patient it blunders with, it has comforted several others.[8]

The forced marriage

The communist victory in 1949 presented both types of doctor with new problems. Traditional doctors were suspect, as their practice relied on a philosophy of China's feudal past; while modern doctors were criticised for their dependence on Western literature and their elitist training. The authorities attempted to force the two schools together and to create a new medical practice unique to China.

Chairman Mao Tse-Tung had given China's medical situation a great deal of thought. In 1944 he cited the following example:

Among the 1,500,000 people of the Shensi-Kangsu-Ningsia Border Region, there are more than 1,000,000 illiterates, there are 2,000 practitioners of witchcraft, and the broad masses are still under the influence of superstition . . . the human and animal mortality rates are both very high . . . In such circumstances, to rely solely on modern doctors is no solution. Of course, modern doctors have advantages over doctors of the old type, but if they do not concern themselves with the sufferings of the people, do not unite with the thousand and more doctors and veterinarians of the old type in the Border Region and do not help them to make progress, then they will actually be helping the witch doctors . . . There are two principles for the united front: the first is to unite, and the second is to criticize, educate and transform.[9]

Although the Communist radicals planned to modernise China's medical practice, they had become accustomed to using traditional remedies during their long struggle to power; for the Japanese and Kuomintang blockade prevented them from importing modern drugs.[10] Also the actual number of modern doctors in 1949 was pitifully inadequate – a mere 10,000 according to some reports – for a population of 550 million people; whereas there were 500,000 traditional doctors.[11]

From 1949 onwards 'united' clinics or hospitals were organised to foster the new relationship between traditional and modern practices.[12] Patients' fees were pooled to pay the doctors' salaries and other expenses. So traditional doctors were being asked not only to give up their private practice but also to share their fiercely guarded secrets; for they still held the feudal notion, 'You must not crack the vase that holds the rice'. Despite their co-operation, traditional doctors were still excluded from large urban hospitals; they were only made use of in rural areas where there was a desperate shortage of modern doctors. Thus modern medicine was definitely the dominant partner in its 'forced marriage' with traditional medicine.

Naturally, the traditional doctors smarted under the unconcealed contempt of their Western-trained colleagues; but it was not long before they exacted satisfying reprisals. In 1955 the Ministry of Health was attacked for its lack of appreciation of traditional practices. Several senior modern physicians were openly criticised for their overbearing Western attitudes and lack of concern for the mass of their patients. The modern doctor's insistence that he had been trained as an expert irritated the communist authorities; whereas the traditional doctor, persecuted in the past by the intellectuals, was exalted for his lack of demands for status or resources. The Press, while castigating modern doctors, released pictures of the white-bearded venerable traditional doctor – showing that the authorities had adopted a loving care for the neglected popular elements in the old culture.

Those taking a stand against modern medicine remembered the days before the Second World War when the Rockefeller Foundation financed the Peking Union Medical College. Here graduates were automatically recognised by the West, and encouraged to travel to the States for further training. They practised from the large cities and amassed considerable fortunes; in other words they failed to treat the mass of the population in the countryside. Other accusations were thrown at the American adventure into Chinese medicine: the charity patients were subjected to barbarous medical experiments, and the local warlords were offered sanctuary for non-medical reasons when they were under attack.[13]

The compromise

The authorities found a clever way out of the quagmire; they accorded both forms of practice equal status. In 1955, Peking Medical College founded the Chinese Traditional Medical Research Institute; at the same time Shanghai Medical College started the Acupuncture Research Institute. By 1959 twenty-seven similar research centres were funded throughout the country to encourage traditional doctors to undertake scientific research into their work. Meanwhile the most important decision was to appoint traditional practitioners to the staffs of hospitals in the large cities.

Since the 1950s all medical students have to study both modern and traditional medicine. Those students who wish to practise traditional medicine have to study the relevant modern knowledge of anatomy, physiology, and so on; while those who wish to practise modern medicine have to attend lectures on various traditional aspects. Premier Chou en-Lai summed up his administration's attitude: 'Make the Motherland's medical heritage serve socialism.'[14]

Even this approach has not solved the fundamental clash between the two schools of medicine; for doctors of one school pay scant regard to the other once they are qualified.[15] These two attitudes to medicine have not been fused, as their bases of thought and expression are clearly not the same; for instance the very word 'disease' has modern and traditional descriptions which are quite different. The two types of doctor diagnose and assess the treatment of disease in totally different ways.

The fiery nature of the argument between the traditional Chinese and Western schools of medicine will become cooler once it is remembered how their different understandings of disease arose. The traditional texts were written by doctors who were forced to rely on their unaided senses in their examination of patients. They were unaware of the cellular structure of the body, and had none of the modern understanding of the nervous system; they did not possess microscopes or any of the other apparatus so essential to modern medical studies. Nevertheless they made some important observations; a great deal of scientific work has been funded both in China and the West in the past two decades to separate the wheat from the chaff. Those who ignore or are unable to understand this scientific work and prefer to accept all the traditional Chinese medical concepts as being utterly true are as blind as those who reject them totally without first studying the evidence.

Part Two

Traditional Acupuncture

In the days before history was recorded in China it is thought that medicine was practised by goatherds who discovered that sharp pieces of flint could be used to relieve various illnesses; they may also have set fire to herbs and deliberately burnt the skin to achieve the same effect.

Some of the earliest writings in China describe a system based on these early observations. Here philosophers who were interested in man's place in the universe described how the same laws they saw governing the world around them determined man's health. Indeed, they concentrated on keeping people healthy wherever this was possible. When a person actually became ill, then the most solemn discourse on the possible causes were described in great detail in elegant books that may have been written as long ago as the second or third centuries BC.

As 90 per cent of acupuncturists in the world pay lip service at least to these classical or 'traditional' ideas of Chinese medicine, a section is required to introduce them. This section is a salute, albeit an incomplete one, to the immense scholarship of these early medical explorers. I have only outlined some of the traditional thoughts and practices here, as in the past three decades there has been a steady growth of work undertaken by doctors of quite a different school – in fact those who are trained in Western medical methods. These doctors are investigating acupuncture in a scientific manner and are developing the subject in directions which are considered in Part Three of this book.

Indeed those readers trained in modern medicine will find Part Three more to their taste as it discusses acupuncture in terms of the discoveries made in the West.

Many people consider that the two schools of acupuncture – traditional and modern – are mutually incompatible. In a superficial sense this is correct; however, we should not ignore the written records of two and a half millennia. I think it is worthwhile for those brought up in modern Western methods to try to understand what the ancient Chinese descriptions were actually intended to mean. Indeed, those who wrote the classical texts may have been amazed to think that anyone would wish to read their words 2,500 years later; they would certainly expect the reader to try his hardest to read between the lines, to see the patient standing before his physician and to understand what went through his mind.

2
Traditional Acupuncture

◆

How did the Chinese look at medicine many years ago? We are lucky to have an early and much quoted manuscript – a *Classic of Internal Medicine*. It is believed that this was written during the tumultuous years of the Warring States period of China (475–221 BC). During these times the ancient feudal system was restructured by almost incessant war between various factions. The outcome was a more sophisticated society less dependent upon local 'gentry'. Power began to lie in the hands of princes, while educated sons of noble rank, dispossessed of their lands by war, had to live by their own exertions. Those who had talent for innovation were called to advise their monarchs, who were only too anxious to enrich and protect their states.

Marked improvements occurred in irrigation, intensive agriculture, fortifications, road building, metallurgy and medicine.[1] Indeed, the advances in metalworking allowed needles to be used in medicine. A passage taken from the *Classic of Internal Medicine* tells us: 'We govern the people, we wish they would not have to take drugs that may be poisonous, nor do we want them to use rough and unrefined stone flints. We should provide them with fine, delicate metal needles.'

The *Classic of Internal Medicine*
In order to increase the reader's respect, the *Classic of Internal*

Medicine was supposed to have been written by a much-worshipped figure who reigned at an earlier date – 2600 BC. He was the Yellow Emperor or Huang Ti himself. 'In ancient times when the Yellow Emperor was born he was endowed with divine talents; while yet in early infancy he could speak; while still very young he was quick of apprehension and penetrating; when he was grown up he was sincere and comprehending; when he was perfect he ascended to Heaven.'[2]

The book describes a conversation between this great man and his royal physician Ch'i Po, as he tried to discover what he could about disease.

The Yellow Emperor wanted to be sure that he could transmit to his sons and grandsons the secrets of medicine and make them known to posterity. He swore that he would not make reckless use of such information.[3] He asked his physician to decipher nature to the utmost degree and explain how disease occurred and how it could be treated. 'One should make public on tablets of jade that which was hidden and sealed in treasuries and store houses, to study it from early dawn until night, and thus make known the precious mechanisms of the Universe.'[4]

These quotations are taken from a remarkable translation in 1972 of the *Classic of Internal Medicine* by Dr Ilza Veith[5] of California University. Her English prose is majestic, giving a flavour of what it must have been like to be a doctor in those days trying to make a sensible system of medicine that could be taught and practised by his pupils.

However, she had numerous difficulties in carrying out her translation; for instance the work was totally unpunctuated. Indeed, the authors of those days sometimes tried to be as obscure as possible to protect their work from being exploited by those of inferior learning.[6] Their intention was to reach out to readers of similar culture to develop a more enlightened understanding of the subject. It must have been a notable feat to have been able to work through passages which were often repeated in subtly different ways to create different effects and some of which were deliberately written in a confusing manner.

The original work was of enormous length. Although it

was written in a philosophical manner to encourage doctors to develop a broader and more enlightened view of their art, the *Classic of Internal Medicine* has become a textbook for many traditional practitioners.

Here we find the thoughts of the legendary Yellow Emperor. He believed that a perfect body was the utmost desire of everyone – 'Man lives on the breath of Heaven and Earth and he achieves perfection through the laws of four seasons.' He felt the whole weight of nature conspiring to produce mankind – 'Covered by heaven, supported by earth, all creation together in its most complete perfection is planned for the greatest achievement: man.'[7] He thanked his physician for so ably explaining how man responded to yin and yang, the two principles in nature.[8]

Yin and yang

Those not brought up in the culture of the ancient philosophers of China find it impossible to fully understand the subtle use of the words *yin* and *yang*.[9]

Crudely one could define them as opposite forces in nature: female (yin) as opposed to male (yang); negative (yin) as opposed to positive (yang).

The Yellow Emperor believed that the principle of yin and yang was the basic principle of the entire universe; it was the principle of everything in creation; it brought about the transformation to parenthood; it was the root and source of life and death.

The most important idea from a doctor's point of view was the fact that heaven and the light from the sky constituted yang; while things of the earth, particularly those lying in the depths of a body, had a yin quality. Anything that had a hot or fiery nature such as the heat of the sun had a yang composition; while anything deeply placed, dark, moist and of a watery nature represented yin.[10]

The Chinese should be praised for appreciating how the products of nature are held together by forces of opposite polarities. Today, the whole of modern physics and chemistry would become unintelligible without a theoretical understanding of negative and positive forces that help to hold matter together.

More was implied: even in an object such as the moon itself, which appeared to be almost entirely yin, a little yang could be found. Conversely the most yang-like object, perhaps the sun, contained a small portion of yin.

As far as medicine was concerned yin and yang had to be present in appropriate quantities in each organ; too much of either contributed to illness. The idea that there are three states (too little, too much and just right) is also present in modern medical thought: for instance, a patient must have a normally functioning thyroid gland to be healthy; too little or too much activity in that gland would cause a *hypo-* or *hyper*thyroid state.

Anyone wishing to use the yin and yang analogy in modern medicine would not have much difficulty in doing so; but, as we shall see, scientists prefer to discuss the functions of the body in terms that do not require so philosophical a concept.

Nevertheless we are entitled to ask how yin and yang ideas helped Chinese physicians.

Yin and yang in medicine
The yin and yang principles were even employed by Chinese anatomists. Like some of their modern counterparts they attempted to explain anatomy in a functional manner which not only helped them arrive at a diagnosis but also assisted in deciding the 'correct' treatment.

They imagined a subject standing to attention, with his back to the sun. Those outer surfaces of the body which were bathed in sunlight were called yang; while those which were shaded or hidden from the sun were yin. There were in fact various subdivisions of the yin and yang surfaces.

In our model of a subject standing in this way, those surfaces of the legs and arms burnt by the sun were called Great Yang; the surfaces that lie along the sides of the limbs were named Lesser Yang; while those surfaces nearer the front that were pleasantly warmed by the sun were referred to as Sunlight Yang (see Figure 2).

Meanwhile, those surfaces on the insides of the arms and legs were also divided into sections: those at the rear were called Lesser Yin; those lying in the middle aspects of the

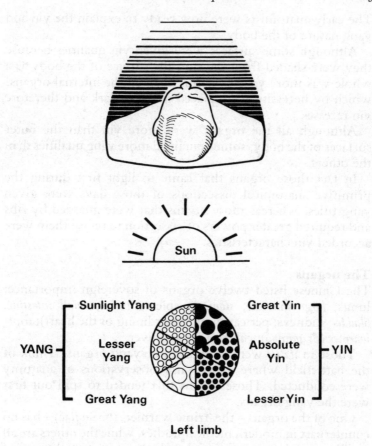

Figure 2   *The yin and yang surfaces of the upper and lower limbs on the left side of the body.*

limbs were Absolute Yin; while those at the front of the shaded surface of the limbs were Great Yin.

A further subdivision was considered necessary: those surfaces that lay on the upper limb were called hand surfaces; whereas those that lay on the leg were called foot surfaces. Thus a pain felt at the outer aspect of the elbow might be referred to as lying within the Lesser Yang of the hand; while the outer aspect of the knee was placed in the province of Sunlight Yang of the foot.

The early anatomists were now ready to explain the yin and yang nature of the body.

Although some surfaces were given yin qualities because they were shaded from the sun, the surface of the body as a whole was more yang in nature than all the internal organs, which by necessity were placed in deep, dark and therefore yin recesses.

Although all the organs were more yin than the outer surfaces of the body, some contained more yang qualities than the others.

In fact those organs that came to light first during the primitive anatomical dissections of those days were given yang titles, whereas those organs that were guarded by ribs and required greater powers of dissection to reveal them were accorded yin characteristics.

The organs

The Chinese listed twelve organs of sovereign importance: lungs; *large intestine*; *stomach*; spleen; heart; *small intestine*; *bladder*; kidneys; pericardium (outer lining of the heart); *triple warmer* (or *sanjiao*); *gall bladder*; and liver.

Those in *italics* were thought to be yang organs. Think of the battlefield where many early observations of anatomy were conducted. Those organs that tended to spill out first were the yang organs.

One of the organs – the 'triple warmer' (or *sanjiao*) – has no counterpart in modern medical studies, while the others are all well known. It is interesting that the most protected organ of all – the brain – was not considered to be an important organ; it was in fact described as being a vital part of bone marrow.

Subdivisions of the organs

We now come to a difficult concept that helped physicians remember in which particular categories of yin and yang the organs were placed.

In the *Classic of Internal Medicine* the royal physician, Ch'i Po, described a remarkable symbolic model.[11]

He tells his reader to imagine the surface of a road. There is a hole in this road leading down to an underground cavern whose roof just touches the road above and whose floor contains an underground stream. The opening of the hole is in fact lined with some special material and is guarded by a hatch cover. Imagine removing the hatch cover and descending into a passage that enters this cavern through an archway.

We can now explain the flow of contact through the various subdivisions of yin and yang. The road and the materials surrounding and guarding the opening into the passage are all bathed in sunlight and are therefore yang surfaces. In fact the road itself is Great Yang, the materials used to line the opening are Lesser Yang and the hatch cover over the hole is Sunlight Yang (see Figure 3).

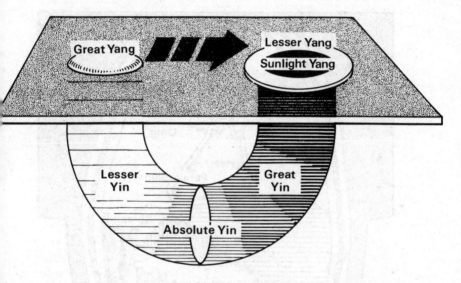

Figure 3   *The flow of 'energy' from yin to yang as explained by the Yellow Emperor's physician.*

The remaining hidden structures are yin: the passageway from the hole to the entrance of the cavern is Great Yin; the archway leading to the cavern is Absolute Yin; while the cavern itself is Lesser Yin.

We can now see how Great Yang passes over Lesser Yang and Sunlight Yang to reach various depths below: first Great Yin, then through Absolute Yin to re-emerge via Lesser Yin. The various categories of the surfaces of the body were arranged in just the same order around the limbs (see Figure 2). This circle or flow of contact through the various surfaces also helped to explain how the organs were arranged in various subdivisions.

A beautifully carved Japanese boxwood model – standing approximately 8 centimetres high – gives us an idea of the shapes the internal organs were considered to be (see Plate 1). For comparison, Western drawings (Figures 4 and 5) show the shapes of these organs as we understand them nowadays from modern anatomical studies; the 'triple warmer' or *sanjiao* is not included as it does not exist.

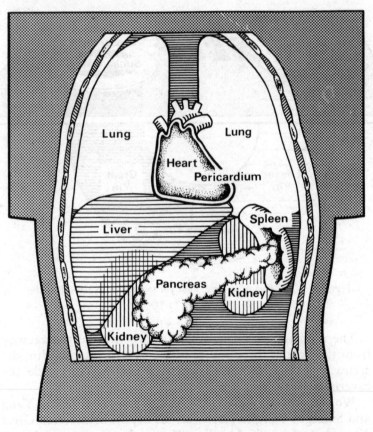

Figure 4   *Modern anatomical drawing of the yin organs, all of which are guarded by the rib cage.*

Lesser Yin organs: heart and kidneys

Lesser Yin organs had to have two qualities: they needed to contain underground springs or, in Ch'i Po's words, 'all that flows rapidly'. At the same time, although deeply placed in the body they had to have direct contact with the outside surface – just as the Lesser Yin cave roof touched the Great Yang surface of the road.

The two organs that have this quality are the *heart* and *kidneys*. Both are concerned with flowing fluids and both are sited in part superficially within the body.

The heart lies solidly in the centre of the chest; yet parts of it can be felt quite superficially on the left side of the chest.

Although for the most part the kidneys lie deep in the body,

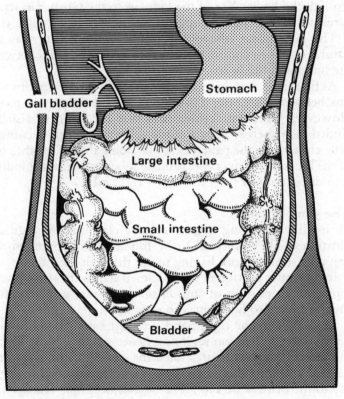

Figure 5   *The yang organs revealed in a modern manner.*

protected by ribs, their lower poles are unprotected and lie perilously close to the surface of the back.

Great Yin organs: lungs and spleen

The Great Yin structures were considered to be 'The foundation of everything that is hidden, mysterious and empty'. In the Chinese mind at least the *lungs* and *spleen* fulfilled this role.

In traditional Chinese anatomy of the spleen it was thought to be indivisible from the pancreas, which was regarded as a tail issuing forth from its depth, passing across to the duodenum, which incidentally was probably incorporated into the traditional concept of the stomach.

Absolute Yin organs: pericardium and liver

To link the Lesser Yin of the kidneys to the Great Yin structures we have to pass through Absolute Yin (see Figure 3).

The *pericardium* (the outer lining of the heart) was the natural organ to choose for this role as it clearly lies between the lungs and the heart (see Figure 4).

At first sight the Chinese choice of the *liver* is not an obvious link between the Lesser Yin kidneys and the Great Yin spleen. However, when one remembers that the Chinese also included the pancreas as part of the spleen, then this becomes a little clearer; for the pancreas at one point almost touches one of the lobes of the liver (the caudate lobe) and the right kidney is in direct contact with the liver's right lobe.

The yang organs

Meanwhile the yang organs require clarification. Figure 5 illustrates. They were all to be found in the abdomen and could be seen without having to cut through the ribs.

In the upper portion of the abdomen stands the *stomach* with a prominent portion of *large intestine* hanging just beneath – these were called Sunlight Yang organs.

Tucked in to the right-hand side is the *gall bladder*, diving deeply into hidden yin regions – hence a Lesser Yang organ; the Lesser Yang structures lined the orifice of the Great Yin passage and were thought to be the 'foundation and bringer of life to the orifices of Yin'. The *Sanjiao* or *Triple Warmer* was also considered to be a Lesser Yang organ.

Spilling over the rest of the abdomen in the upper portion of the pelvis were the Great Yang (or the 'Great Thoroughfare') organs – the *small intestine* and *bladder*.

The various categories of yin and yang and their organs can now be summarised in Table 1.

Table 1   *Various yin and yang categories of the organs*

YIN	column 1	column 2
Great Yin	LUNGS	SPLEEN
Absolute Yin	PERICARDIUM	LIVER
Lesser Yin	HEART	KIDNEYS
YANG		
Great Yang	SMALL INTESTINE	BLADDER
Lesser Yang	TRIPLE WARMER	GALL BLADDER
Sunlight Yang	LARGE INTESTINE	STOMACH

Connections between the organs and body surfaces

An essential and rather remarkable part of Chinese medical thought was the idea that each organ had a special relationship with various parts of the body surface according to the yin and yang categories that have just been described. Thus a Great Yin organ, for example, was intimately connected with a Great Yin area of the body's surface.

Table 1, however, shows us that each category (Great Yin, Absolute Yin, etc.) was represented not by one but two organs. In each pair, the organ that was thought to lie at a higher level (or to be more prominently displayed) in the body has been placed in column 1; these organs were related to a *hand* surface while its fellow (column 2) was thought to be connected to a *foot* surface.

Table 2 tells us which category of body surface – *hand* or *foot* – was connected to which organ.

How were the organs and their related surfaces linked? A complicated network of vessels or channels, called *meridians*, is described in greater detail in Chapter 3. Each category of body surface had its own named tributaries of this system.

Although there were meant to be no less than five types of meridians, perhaps the most important were called *main meridians*. Each main meridian was named after the particular category of the body surface it lay in; thus Sunlight Yang surfaces had Sunlight Yang main meridians.

Table 2 *The organs and their related surfaces*

YIN SURFACES		*Organs*
Great Yin	hand	LUNG
Great Yin	foot	SPLEEN
Absolute Yin	hand	PERICARDIUM
Absolute Yin	foot	LIVER
Lesser Yin	hand	HEART
Lesser Yin	foot	KIDNEYS
YANG SURFACES		*Organs*
Great Yang	hand	SMALL INTESTINE
Great Yang	foot	BLADDER
Lesser Yang	hand	TRIPLE WARMER
Lesser Yang	foot	GALL BLADDER
Sunlight Yang	hand	LARGE INTESTINE
Sunlight Yang	foot	STOMACH

As will be explained later, each organ was supposed to be connected directly to its appropriate main meridian: the liver, for example, was therefore linked to the *foot Absolute Yin* main meridian (see Table 2). In many modern textbooks describing acupuncture, perhaps in an attempt to simplify matters, the foot Absolute Yin main meridian is called the *liver meridian*.

Chi or 'energy'
The prime function of the organs and meridians was to supply a 'life force' called *chi* (pronounced as the first four letters of *chee*se) to all parts of the body. It is probably easier for a lay person than for a scientist to imagine what the Chinese really meant by this term.

Perhaps the best English translation of *chi* is the word 'energy' in the oldest sense of the word. When a patient feels ill he has 'no energy'; as soon as he recovers he feels his 'energy' returning.

Here we are not discussing the physicists' use of the word which was first employed in 1807 to describe a body's power of doing work. Rather we are thinking of a person's qualities of vigour or intensity of speech and action.

The Chinese refused to make a clear distinction between 'spirit' and 'matter'.

The manner in which they described their ideas about *chi* was that of a poet or philosopher rather than a physicist. Perhaps the best description was given by a biologist in Ming times as late as the fourteenth century AD.[12] Here he described how the rain, dew, frost and snow had subtle spirits or *chi*; but he drew the distinction that these spirits were quite devoid of endowments or sensitivity.

Other substances such as herbs, wood and some minerals were thought to possess another type of *chi* which allowed them to preserve their form and shape but did not give them any sensitivity. Whilst the *chi* of birds, beasts, insects and fishes preserved not only their form but also gave them sensitivity. He even paused to state that different parts of these creatures had different forms of *chi*: for instance their feathers, fur and scales had shape without sensitivity; whilst their excretions and watery secretions had *chi* of the type similar to that supposed to exist in rain, dew and frost.

Drs Joseph Needham and Lu Gwei-Djen of Cambridge University have spent the last two decades translating and interpreting the history of Chinese science.[13] On the mysterious question of *chi*, they considered that, from a Chinese point of view, it was an infinitely vaporous substance which could be regarded as having non-material radiations which today could be called radio waves, X-rays or other non-particulate energies. Or it could be more substantial and appear in a gaseous state resembling air.[14]

Of course high frequency energy was quite unknown and it was not until the 1840s that physicists recognised the same forms underlying dynamic, thermal, gravitational, optical and electrical changes. Was this the same phenomenon imagined by Chinese philosophers? 'It is pure *chi* which changes the myriad things; where it agglomerates it causes life; where it disperses it causes death. What has never been aggregated or dispersed has never been alive or dead. The guests (living things or phenomena) come and go, but their material basis remains unchanged.' Drs Joseph Needham and Lu Gwei-Djen ask whether this was a premonition of atomic materialism where all changes are only apparent, the fundamental particles themselves remaining unchanged but taking part in ever-changing combinations.

Whatever the real ideas about *chi* were, the Chinese felt that it had to permeate the substance of the body to enliven the internal organs and limbs.

Yet the organs themselves could influence the flow of *chi* round the body. In other words, *chi* circulated through the organs and received some influence from each one during its passage; the organs themselves could be damaged if an insufficient quantity or the wrong sort of *chi* reached them.[15] This was a remarkable insight into medicine; the organs do rely on the correct circulation of various substances for their proper function; yet a damaged organ might well interfere with the normal circulation of such substances to the rest of the body.

Chi had both yin and yang elements which were apparently at least partly under the control of the organs; indeed, *chi* flowed through an elaborate system of channels or meridians between the organs to allow them to achieve a perfect 'mix'. When this had been achieved then the meridians could conduct *chi* to the outermost parts of the body to maintain their functions.

Our next question, therefore, is: How did the meridians achieve this remarkable feat?

3
Meridians and the Causes of Disease

◆

Meridians
The word 'meridian' implies a geographical term – the great circle of a celestial sphere – while here it was meant to be a *chi*-conducting vessel or channel taking an irregular course through the body at various depths; yet the word 'meridian' has caught the imagination and will be used in the rest of this book.

Meridians were supposed to be divided into five groups; these were main, connecting or *lo*, divergent, muscle, and extra meridians. They all served different functions.

Main meridians
As has already been said, each organ was thought to be connected to a particular part of the body surface; for instance, the liver was connected to the *foot Absolute Yin* surface. Each of these surfaces had its own main meridian. At some point along its length it was supposed to be connected by a branch to its associated organ.

Each organ had in fact two main meridians – one on each side of the body.

Yin and yang main meridians were linked together in pairs by connecting or *lo* meridians (described later). At first sight the pairs that were chosen for this purpose appear strange bedfellows: Sunlight Yang with Great Yin; Lesser Yang with Absolute Yin; and Great Yang with Lesser Yin.

Yet referring back to Chi Po's symbolic model (Figure 3, page 25) makes all apparently clear: the nearest yin portion beneath the Sunlight Yang 'hatchway' is the Great Yin passage; the Lesser Yang and Absolute Yin both link sub-divisions of the same polarity; finally, immediately below the surface of the Great Yang road surface is the Lesser Yin cave.

The pairs of meridians are shown in Table 3, and they are referred to again and again in the traditional literature. Often one organ of a pair would be confused with the other.[1]

An almost poetical symmetry can be seen in the order of surfaces and their related organs as laid out in the following pairs:

Table 3 *Paired organs and their related surfaces*

Pairs		Surfaces	Organs
Sunlight Yang/	1	hand Great Yin	LUNG
Great Yin		hand Sunlight Yang	LARGE INTESTINE
	2	foot Sunlight Yang	STOMACH
		foot Great Yin	SPLEEN
Great Yang/	3	hand Lesser Yin	HEART
Lesser Yin		hand Great Yang	SMALL INTESTINE
	4	foot Great Yang	BLADDER
		foot Lesser Yin	KIDNEYS
Lesser Yang/	5	hand Absolute Yin	PERICARDIUM
Absolute Yin		hand Lesser Yang	TRIPLE WARMER
	6	foot Lesser Yang	GALL BLADDER
		foot Absolute Yin	LIVER

Chi was thought to flow from one main meridian to another in the order shown in the right-hand column of Table 3 from the lungs at the beginning of the cycle through large intestine, stomach, spleen, heart, small intestine, bladder, kidney, pericardium, triple warmer, gall bladder, liver and around again (see Figure 6). A complete cycle occurred twenty-five times during the day and twenty-five times during the night.

The order of main meridians shown in Figure 6 is the one

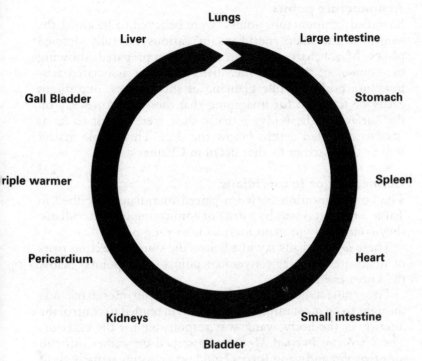

Figure 6 *Circulation of* chi *through the main meridians.*

used in almost all Chinese textbooks. Even in English translations they rarely appear to be arranged in alphabetical order in the text.

Careful study of the courses of these main meridians shows that all six yang channels met in the head, while the six yin meridians met in the chest region close to the shoulder. The lack of yin main meridians in the head had to be overcome by other types of meridians yet to be described.

Chi flowed upwards into the head along the hand yang vessels; meanwhile the foot yang main meridians conducted *chi* down from the head towards the lower extremities.

The opposite arrangement took place in the yin main meridians: *chi* passed from the chest towards the upper limbs in the hand yin channels; but the foot yin main meridians directed *chi* upwards from the feet to the chest.

Acupuncture points

So-called 'acupuncture points' were believed to lie along the length of the main meridians in various carefully defined places. Many charts and atlases have been prepared, showing the courses of the main meridians and their associated acupuncture points. While glancing at such atlases, one might easily be forgiven for imagining that these structures lay on the surface of the body; actually they were meant to lie at various recorded depths below the skin. This whole matter will be discussed in further detail in Chapter 7.

Connecting or *lo* meridians

The communication between paired meridians described in Table 3 (page 34) was by virtue of connecting or *lo* meridians: they connected yin main meridians to yang ones.

These *lo* meridians lay just below the skin connecting pairs of main meridians at convenient points (or *lo* points) below the knees and elbows.

This contact between yin and yang main meridians was thought to be most important. While yin tended to control the interior of the body, yang was responsible for the exterior. The *Classic of Internal Medicine* described the rather difficult idea that yin and yang forces could on occasion actually fight each other to the detriment of the patient:

> When serious changes occur in Yang, death ensues, and when they occur in Yin death also ensues, because then Yin and Yang oppose each other. For in regard to medical treatment one must also take into consideration that two forces in nature can attack each other on unusual occasions and even at regular occurrences.[2]

Lo meridians acted as sluices to maintain harmony between the two.

The nearest equivalent to the idea of *lo* meridians from a Western point of view would be small vessels such as capillaries forming a vital link between small arteries and veins.[3]

Divergent meridians

Another important but complex system for linking pairs of

organs and their main meridians was thought to exist: structures called divergent meridians dived deeply into the body from points on their parent main meridians (above the knees and elbows); each named divergent meridian found its way through the tissues to connect directly with the other organ of the same pair. As can be seen from Table 3 (page 34), the heart divergent meridian was attached in this way to the small intestine.

Having contacted their relevant organs, the divergent meridians proceeded upwards through the body in pairs to emerge in the neck region. Here both yin and yang divergent meridians were connected together to the yang member of the paired main meridians passing through the neck.

To continue our example of the heart divergent meridian, it passed down from the heart main meridian from a point above the elbow to attach itself to the small intestine; from there it travelled upwards to the neck to merge with the small intestine main meridian.

The divergent meridians played an important role: they allowed yin organs to influence the head region; for no yin main meridians proceeded further than the chest.

Muscle meridians
The muscles and joints apparently required a set of meridians also; these were called muscle meridians. *Chi* flowed through all of these from the fingers and toes towards the body.

The three yin muscle meridians from the upper limb met in the chest; while the three yin muscle meridians from the legs united in the genitalia.

The three yang muscle meridians of the arm converged on each other at the side of the head; the three yang muscle meridians of the leg came together on the cheek.

Although the muscle meridians took their names from the nearest main meridians, they were not considered to be connected to the relevant organs. They were merely involved in diseases affecting bones and joints.

Extra meridians
Eight further or 'extra' meridians were described.[4] They were very similar in many ways to the main meridians, although

not one was directly linked to the internal organs; furthermore, six of them had no acupuncture points of their own.
Apparently these linked points which already existed in other
meridians. Together the extra meridians acted as a 'reservoir'
to maintain the pressure of *chi* in the main meridians.

Two of the extra meridians were given acupuncture points
of their own: one of these, the *Conception Vessel*, conveyed *chi*
up the midline of the front of the body from the groin to the
chin; while the other, the *Governing Vessel*, transported *chi* up
the midline of the back from the tip of the coccyx (or tail bone)
over the back of the head and down the centre of the face as far
as the upper lip (see Figures 7 and 8).

Why were the meridians ever thought of?

To try to understand why Chinese doctors were so concerned
about meridians, we have to think what it was like to be a
doctor in those days. They had little knowledge of the
nervous system and did not, so far as we know, realise that the
body was composed of individual cells linked together by the
circulation of various fluids (including blood) and the nervous
system. However, they did realise that the circulation of
blood was vitally important and even the *Classic of Internal
Medicine* described blood passing through organs. These
aspects are discussed again in Chapter 10.

They were unaware that as far as the nervous system is
concerned the body may be divided into various segments (see
Figure 9). This segmental pattern follows an altogether
different picture from that presented by meridians. Nevertheless enormous trouble was taken to trace out the paths of the
main meridians on wooden, ivory, papier mâché and bronze
statues varying in height from life-size to a few centimetres
(see Plate 2).

Numerous drawings and fine paintings were made to illustrate the paths of meridians. Most modern textbooks on the
subject show only the courses of the main meridians, but
many works written in the 1960s or earlier described all five
types of meridians in considerable detail. Dr Felix Mann's
excellent book, *The Meridians of Acupuncture*,[5] gives not only
very useful drawings of each type of meridian derived from

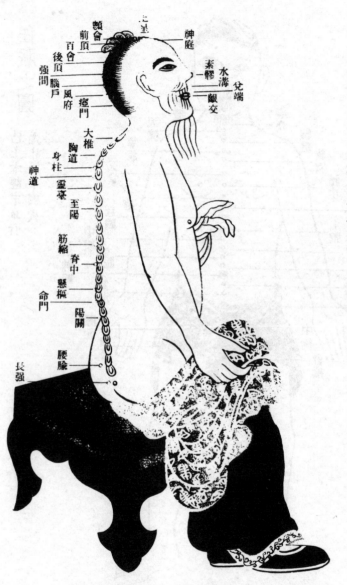

督脈之圖

已上本經中行單

穴計二十七穴

囟會
頂會
前頂
百會
後頂
強間
腦戶
風府
瘖門
大椎
胸道
身柱
靈臺
至陽
筋縮
脊中
懸樞
陽關
腰腧
長強
神道
命門

神庭
素髎
水溝
齗交
兌端

圖六十八——仿明版古圖（十四）

Figure 7　*Ming dynasty drawing of the Governing Vessel.*

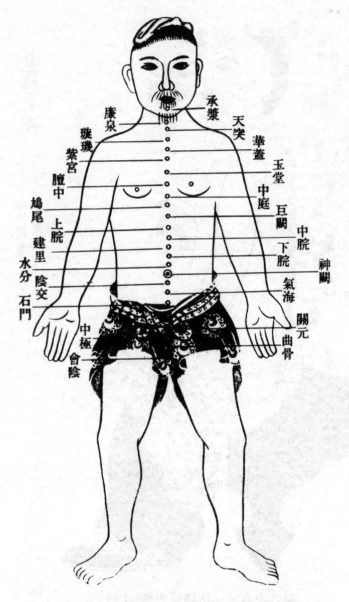

任脈之圖 巳上本經中單行
穴計二十四穴

承漿
康泉
琁璣
紫宮
膻中
鳩尾
建里
水分
石門

天突
華蓋
玉堂
中庭
巨闕
中脘
下脘
氣海
關元
曲骨

上脘
陰交

神闕

中極
會陰

圖六十七——仿明版古圖(十三)

Figure 8   *Ming dynasty drawing of the Conception Vessel.*

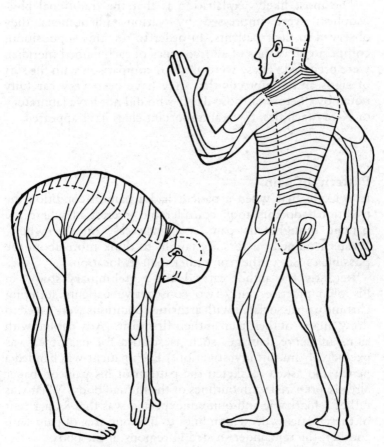

Figure 9 *The body divided into segments according to modern studies of the distribution of nerves to the skin.*

some of these earlier sources,[6,7] but also gives a lucid description of their supposed pathways and functions.

We have still not been able to answer *why* the Chinese scholars considered the meridians and their positions within the body to be so important, particularly as we in the West have not seen any sensible evidence of their existence. Indeed, the modern Chinese anatomists have not found any supporting evidence either.

The most likely explanation is that the traditional philosophers were impressed by various phenomena they
observed in their patients. In order to test this supposition,
composite drawings of all five types of each named meridian
were prepared. These were used for comparison with the sort
of signs and symptoms that may have been very carefully
noted by doctors of those days, who did not have laboratory
or X-ray facilities. Several important clues have appeared.

Patterns of pain

It is likely that when a patient had a painful condition the
traditional doctors took considerable interest in where the
patient thought his pain was; whereas, on the whole,
Western-trained doctors are taught to think more about the
possible causes of the pain rather than its location.

Recently the author carried out a preliminary study[8] in
his own practice. Fifty-two consecutive patients suffering
chronic pain associated with arthritic conditions were asked to
draw 'maps' of their pain at their first visit. (Any patient with
signs of nerve damage, such as sciatica for example, was
excluded from this investigation.) Each patient was handed a
pencil and asked to sketch the pattern of his pain on paper
already prepared with outlines of the human body. What was
rather remarkable and quite unexpected was that 85 per cent
of these patients drew thin lines to link one area of pain with
another; the remainder shaded in regions of the body.

Ninety-six per cent of these thin lines required only one
meridian to explain them. A typical example is shown in
Figure 10. In fact, only 31 per cent of these lines lay within one
nerve segment. In other words, amongst these patients, at
least, there was a strong tendency for the distribution of their
pains to flow along the paths of meridians rather than be
confined to the boundaries of nerve segments. Further studies
of this kind are needed to confirm this phenomenon.

If there is a connection between patterns of pain and meridians, the simplest explanation is that the Chinese may have
based their meridian charts on numerous patients' descriptions of their aches and pains.

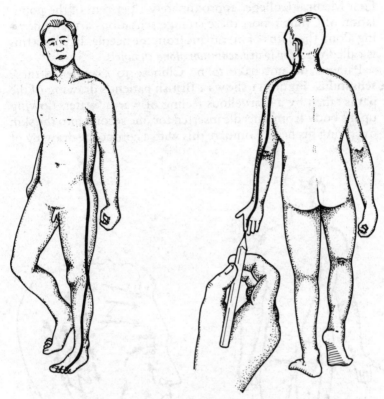

Figure 10   *Examples of meridian-like patterns of pain drawn by a patient on an outline of the human body.*

Sensations produced by acupuncture

Dramatic events sometimes follow the insertion of a needle. As will be explained in Chapter 14, the Chinese often quite deliberately insert their needles to a required depth within muscles or other tissues to produce bizarre or unpleasant sensations called *techi*. Patients may say with some surprise that they have unusual sensations radiating away from the site of the needle – 'Good heavens, I can feel warmth flowing up my leg from that needle in my foot!'

According to Professor Cao Xiao-Ding, Head of the Research Department of Acupuncture Analgesia and Deputy Director of the Institute of Basic Medical Science at Shanghai

First Medical College, approximately 1 per cent of the population of China report these strange sensations actually flowing along the paths of meridians from the needle. In China this is called the *propagated sensation along channels*.

Patients do not have to be Chinese to experience these sensations. Figure 11 shows a British patient's drawing of the paths taken by a marvellous feeling of warm 'water' flowing up his body from a needle inserted for one second into the skin overlying his heel. Compare this with a composite drawing of

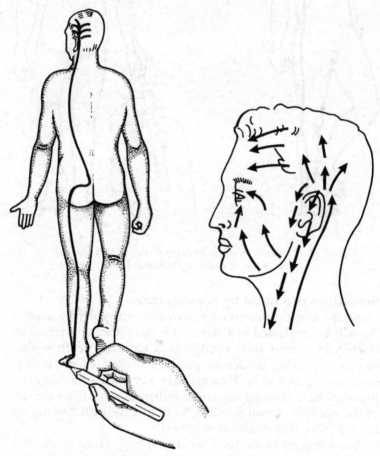

Figure 11   *Pattern of sensation drawn by a patient on an outline of the body following the insertion of a needle in his heel.*

all five types of foot Great Yang or bladder meridians[9] (Figure 12). This particular patient had a rare and remarkable facility for describing the courses of channels found only in Chinese sources, whenever a needle was inserted. He produced a faithful account of meridians on numerous occasions and never seemed to make a mistake.

It is possible that at least some of the early 'authorities' on meridians in the early days had this gift also. They would be able to map their own sensations with comparative ease by merely inserting a needle into their own bodies and recording their experiences.

It is important to note that the fact that a sensation takes place along a certain pathway does *not* necessarily imply that

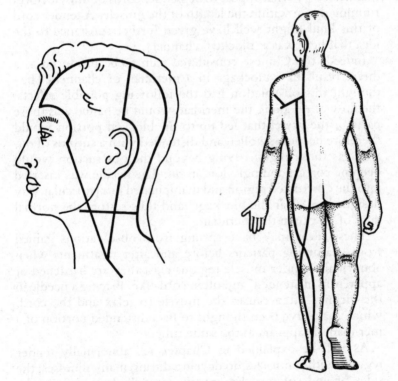

Figure 12 *Composite drawing of the bladder meridians taken from several traditional Chinese sources, which compares interestingly with the patient's drawing in Figure 11.*

there is a physical structure such as a vessel or channel running in the same direction. There are more than enough connections within the central nervous system to account for such experiences. Indeed, the Chinese have found that these sensations can be elicited in 'phantom' limbs (where patients who have had amputated limbs still feel their presence); here no structures of any kind exist.

Tender muscles
In many patients suffering chronic pain, careful examination reveals exquisitely tender regions within muscles. These usually appear as nodules or hardened 'lumps' within the body of an otherwise relaxed muscle; frequently, however, they are manifested by what appear to be slender cords of muscle fibres running down within the length of the muscle. A tender cord of this kind might well have given further substance to the idea that here was a 'blocked' channel.

Indeed, the Chinese considered pain to be produced as a direct result of a blockage in a meridian or channel. They thought this obstruction had the following possible effects: the flow of *chi* along the meridian would be halted and those parts of the vessel that led up to the blocked portion would therefore become swollen and distended with a surplus of *chi*, whereas those regions lying beyond the obstruction would become correspondingly low in *chi*. The needle was inserted into the obstructed region and manipulated in a particular way designed to 'clear the blockage' and thus restore the normal flow of *chi* down the meridian.

These ideas may have sprung from observations gained from examining patients before and after treatment; when abnormally tender muscle regions exist they are hardened or apparently 'distended' and often cord-like. Placing a needle in the vicinity often causes the muscle to relax and the cord, which may have been thought to be a distended portion of a meridian, disappears at the same time.

As will be explained in Chapter 14, abnormally tender regions within muscles do develop during many illnesses; the sides or ends of muscles are the most likely regions to be affected in this way as these are the areas where the blood supply is at its worst. A careful look at a map of meridians prepared in a modern manner (see Figure 13) to show their relationship with muscles and other structures reveals that for most of their courses they connect points lying along the edges or ends of muscles.

Movement patterns

The Chinese took a great deal of interest in therapeutic exercises: doctors prescribed flowing trance-like exercises called

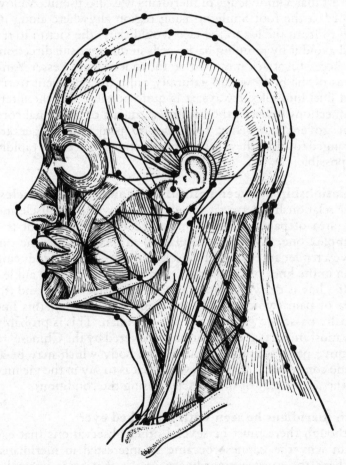

Figure 13 *Distribution of acupuncture points and yang meridians in the head and neck. Note how the points often appear to be at the edge or end of a muscle.*

shadow boxing or *Tai-Chi*. The study of balance and muscle control was considered to be an important part of remaining healthy. Similar discoveries were employed in self-defence or the martial arts.

Although a participant in a martial arts school probably concentrated on learning the 'vital points' where his opponent could be seriously wounded by a blow or small dart (carried concealed in a sleeve), it may have occurred to the masters of the art that a knowledge of meridians was also useful. A blow aimed at the foot Sunlight Yang region anywhere along its length from the leg to the face would cause the victim to try and avoid it by jumping backwards in the opposite direction. A successful attack mounted on the foot or hand Lesser Yang areas of the body would naturally cause the opponent to try and hurl himself sideways; it is quite possible that the interconnections between the various segments of the spinal cord that govern our reflex responses to pain and danger are arranged to allow these protective reactions to occur as rapidly as possible.

Relationship between painful areas and tender muscles
The relationship between a tender region within a muscle and the area of pain actually complained of by the patient is a complex one. As will be explained in Chapter 14, one can have a tender area within a muscle in the hip region producing pain in the knee or sometimes even as far away as the ankle.

If a line is drawn linking the tender muscle region and the area of pain (which is referred from that muscle), this line usually passes down the path of a meridian. This is probably the most important observation discovered by the Chinese: to remove pain, stimulate a part of the body which may be at some considerable distance away (that is to say in the vicinity of the tender part of the muscle causing the condition).

Can meridians be seen with the naked eye?
Although there must be several other observations that explain why the Chinese became so interested in meridians, perhaps the most extraordinary one is that areas normally traversed by the imaginary channels displayed in the acupuncture charts can actually be highlighted on the body and seen

with the naked eye under the following circumstances:[10] the entire body is covered in a reflective substance such as oil or water to make the skin shiny; the person, prepared in this way, poses in positions similar to those found in Ming dynasty (1368–1644) paintings of meridians; provided he stands in a room lit by only one light source, highlights may be seen coursing over the skin along the paths of the meridians (see Plate 4).

Where the surface of the body is relatively flat (for example the back of the hand) a diffusely spread out highlight occurs; but where there is a markedly curved part on cross-section (in the forearm for example) then the highlight becomes a thin line resembling a channel. The reader may check this for himself next time his hand and arm are wet with water in a room lit with only one light source.

As a teaching aid for pupils, the masters of acupuncture probably asked an artist to draw what he could actually see on a body covered in oil, lit by the sun or a single lamp – standing in various positions which they knew would reveal the paths of the meridians in a manner which encompassed all the phenomena they had observed in their patients.

Although there is this remarkable similarity between high-lights seen in this way and early maps of meridians, there is in fact no historical evidence that they were drawn from life as has been suggested here.

The usual explanation
The usual explanation for meridians is that they link well-known acupuncture points with similar functions.

Yet, when one glances at books describing the use of each acupuncture point on a particular meridian, one finds that although there are some similarities there are in fact many startling dissimilarities between the supposed functions of points placed close to each other.

A good example of this may be found in a much quoted modern text book, *An Outline of Chinese Acupuncture*.[11] Two consecutive points on the same meridian were selected at random – *houxi* and *wangu*. These two points lie a centimetre or so apart on the side of the hand on the hand Great Yang or small intestine meridian. Their imagined functions as far as treatment is concerned were described as follows: *houxi* was recommended for stiffness or rigidity of the neck, ringing in the ears, deafness, pain in the back of the head, lumbago, paralysis of the upper limbs, night sweating, epilepsy and malaria; while *wangu* was apparently used for arthritis of the elbow, wrists and finger joints, headache, vomiting, ringing in the ears and gall bladder disease. (It must be said here that such lists of supposed functions of acupuncture points cannot be accepted by most Western-trained doctors; it stretches too far their willingness to try to understand the subject. However, the matter is taken up again in perhaps a more favourable light in Chapter 14.)

Only those meridians which actually link up acupuncture points along their course (the main and extra meridians) can be explained in this way. The remainder – the *lo*, divergent and muscle meridians – presumably require some other explanation.

Blood vessels and meridians

Another possibility is that the meridians were related in some way to blood vessels. Certainly in the ancient texts no clear distinction was made between blood vessels and meridians. Indeed, the yin components of *chi* – whose functions were to nourish the body – were actually believed to be transported in the blood vessels, while the yang component – whose function was to protect – circulated outside the blood vessels between the skin and the flesh. The state of this yang component could apparently be determined by examining the patient's complexion.

Complexion

The colours of the complexion played a vital role in Chinese diagnosis of disease, just as it does in the West today: paleness, greenness, redness, yellowness and blackness of the skin's complexion were all noted in the *Classic of Internal Medicine* in the presence of serious illnesses of various sorts.[12]

Dangerous connections of the meridians

The meridians provided a connection between the internal organs and the outer surfaces of the body. This connection was at some times dangerous, according to the Chinese; for all sorts of harmful agents from the surrounding air could enter them and work their way down to the inside of the body.

This is well described in the *Classic of Internal Medicine* when the Yellow Emperor asked, 'How can one describe the process of falling ill and the changes it brings about?' His physician replied, 'It is the winds and weather (the eight winds) that cause chills and fevers. Diseases arising from overwork cause exhaustion of the diaphragm. Oppressive airs cause madness; constant winds cause inability to retain food, and when abundant winds cause disease within the pulse they bring about sores and ulcers. The transformations and changes wrought by illness cannot be overcome or even enumerated.'[13]

According to the *Classic of Internal Medicine*, the climate had access to the internal organs in the following ways: 'The heavenly climate circulates within the lungs; the winds circulate within the liver; thunder penetrates the heart; the air of a ravine penetrates the stomach; the rain penetrates the kidneys.'

Causes of diseases

Wind, cold, summer heat, damp, dryness and fire were feared as possible causes of disease: wind – or rather 'evil wind' – produced coughing, a runny nose and headache, and could combine with other noxious influences to cause diseases that were called 'wind-cold', 'wind-heat', and so on; cold entered meridians and were thought to provoke fevers to counteract it, together with cramps and pains appearing in muscles, accompanied by diarrhoea and abdominal pain.

Summer heat was blamed for causing fainting, palpitations and a parched mouth. Dampness was accused of being the basis of a variety of ills from a 'melancholic' chest to the vomiting of foul-smelling food.

Dryness, apparently caused sweating, coughing and a dislike of the cold. Fire burnt the lungs and produced blood in the saliva.

Invasions of the climate were thought to be transformed by the viscera into five emotions: joy, anger, sympathy, grief and fear. An excess of any of these emotions could be as damaging as the climate itself: the liver could be damaged by anger; the heart could be injured by joy; the stomach could be overcome by extreme sympathy; the lungs could be overwhelmed by extreme grief; and the kidneys could be mastered by fear.[14]

Those physicians following Chinese traditional medicine worried lest all these evils would lie dormant in the body and appear in another season. Fortunately they believed that none of these meteorological influences could harm the body if the protecting yang element of *chi* (lying outside the blood vessels) was carrying out its role properly:[15] 'When people are quiet and clear, their skin and flesh is closed and protected. Even a heavy storm, afflictions, or poison, cannot injure those people who live in accord with the natural order.'[16]

The effects of food

The meridians were also thought capable of transmitting *flavours* around the body and to each of the viscera: 'We know that the heart craves the bitter flavor; the lungs crave the pungent flavor; the liver craves the sour flavor; the spleen craves the sweet flavor; and the kidneys crave the salty flavor.'[17]

These cravings could be satisfied, however: wheat, mutton, almonds, apricots and scallions could supply the bitter flavour; glutinous yellow panicled millet, chicken meat, peaches and onions could provide the pungent flavour; small peas, dog meat, plums and leeks could add the sour flavour; while large beans, pork, chestnuts and coarse greens could lend a salty flavour.

Yet too much of any particular flavour was considered dangerous:

> Too much salt causes hardening of the pulse and appearance of tears and complexion changes. Too much bitterness causes withering of the skin and falling out of body hair. Too pungent a flavor causes knotting of the muscles and withering of the finger and toe nails. Too much sour flavor causes hardening and wrinkling of the flesh and slack lips. Too much sweetness causes aching in the bones and the hair of the head falls out.

Geographical distribution of disease

It was believed that the regions of China with their different climates and foods caused various diseases to appear.

Those from the east lived near the sea and ate fish and salty food; they suffered from internal burning and ulcers – both of these could be cured by acupuncture. Those from the west had dwellings of stone in fertile lands and ate an excellently varied diet, lived on hillsides and had warm clothing so their bodies were robust and impervious to external diseases; consequently their diseases were of an internal nature and required 'poison' medicines to cure them. Those from the north lived in exposed mountainous regions and had only milk products to sustain them; to treat their diseases borne in by the cold required needles warmed by a process called moxibustion. Those from the south lived in fertile regions with an abundance of sun and dew, and lived on sour foods and curds; they suffered contracted muscles and numbness which could be treated by acupuncture.[18]

The purpose of meridians

The remarkable notion that both the life-giving 'energy' or *chi* on the one hand and destructive forces on the other were conducted in the specific channels or meridians around the body allowed the traditional Chinese physicians not only to explain the cause of diseases but also how to diagnose their yin qualities. This requires further elaboration in Chapter 4, and, as we shall see in Chapters 6 and 7, provided an apparently satisfactory means of treatment in many circumstances.

4
Examining the Pulse

◆

We have already considered how the study of the complexion gave the Chinese doctors an impression of the state of the protective or yang components of *chi*. How then was the yin (or nourishing) element studied?

The yin element of each main meridian was believed to have its own pulse and on many occasions in the original text was described as actually being an artery. (A large amount of blood issuing forth from a wound in the skin would be thought to be coming from one of these main meridians, whereas a small amount of blood would be thought of as coming from one of the *lo* meridians.)

It was believed that all the organs contributed to the quality of pulsation in the arteries; therefore a skilled physician could determine the state of the organs by feeling the pulses in a special way. To feel a normal pulse was a great pleasure: 'When a man is serene and healthy the pulse of the heart flows and connects, just as pearls are joined together or like a string of red jade – then one speaks of a healthy heart.'[1] But when the heart's function was poor, then 'the pulse beats are irregular like a hammer'.[2]

To appreciate the significance of the qualities of a patient's pulse the physician's imagination had to be concentrated on what he knew of the interplay between the organs; for instance, he was taught to believe that the full vigour of the pulses was maintained by the stomach. If the stomach failed in its duties, the splendid proportions of the normal pulse were reduced, exposing the inadequate efforts of the other viscera: 'man uses water and grain as his basis for existence, hence when he is without water and grain he must die. Those pulses which are not reinforced by the stomach merely obtain support from the viscera but not the vital force of the stomach.'[3]

Interpreting the pulse in this way was extraordinarily complicated. The seasons themselves had an influence on the pulse. A physician who was unaware of this might well make the wrong diagnosis: 'In days of spring the pulse is superficial, like wood floating on water, or like a fish gliding through the waves. In summer days the pulse within the skin is drifting and light, and everywhere there is an excess of creation. . . . In winter the torpid insects are all around the bone, quiet and delicate like the nobleman residing in his mansion.'[4] Once the doctor knew the normal seasonal variations, if he detected a pulse that had become discordant with the seasons then he could assume that the patient's viscera were not acting in harmony.

To make matters more complicated, each individual organ's pulse had its own variations. For instance, 'In summer the pulse of the stomach should be like the beats of a fine hammer . . . During the long summer the pulse of the stomach should be soft and feeble . . . In autumn the pulse of the stomach should be small and rough . . . In winter the pulse of the stomach should be small and like a stone.'[5]

The pulses of the three regions of the body
The body was divided into three regions (upper, middle and lower), each of which was divided into three subdivisions – 'heaven', 'earth', and 'man'. Each subdivision had its own artery, whose pulsation the physician could study to discover what was happening there (see Plate 3).

Twelve positions on the radial pulse
The most favoured pulse was the radial pulse of the wrist (representing the heavenly element of the middle region). Each radial artery was examined with three fingers placed side by side; each fingertip occupying approximately one centimetre's length on the artery. The index finger was placed as

near to the wrist as possible over the first 'segment' of the artery; the second finger pressed on the second 'segment'; while the third finger marked the third 'segment'.

The fingers could be used to press lightly or more firmly; therefore each 'segment' could be examined with superficial or deep pressures. Thus *twelve* positions could be found; the total number was composed of a pair of superficial and deep pressure positions in the three 'segments' in the left and right radial arteries. Each of the twelve positions was believed to be under the influence of a particular organ. In other words, the examiner was able to determine the state of each organ in turn by examining the quality of sensations from his fingertips at each position of the radial pulse.

Fierce controversy reigns to this day about which organs influence and occupy which position in the radial pulses. However, all agreed that the yang organs were accorded the superficial sides while the yin organs were placed in the deep positions (see Figure 14).

The positions of the organs on the pulse (see Figure 14) were considered to be very important and were incorporated in various laws of acupuncture which will be explained in some detail later on in Chapter 6. However, modern teaching of traditional acupuncture has rather abandoned these positions and the pupil is taught to examine the pulse as one unfragmented unit.

Twenty-eight varieties of sensation derived from the examination of the abnormal pulse had to be studied and recognised, ten of which are described here:

Fu mo, a light floating pulse, indicated the fact that the 'evil wind' had successfully attacked the yang or external defences; *ch'en mo*, a deep pulse as if the vessel had actually sunk into the bone, indicated a 'dormant' *chi* disturbance deep in the yin interior of the body; *shu mo*, a rapid yang pulse (six beats to each breath), indicated heat in the body usually accompanied by a dry mouth, constipation and diminished urine output; *hua mo*, a slippery pulse 'like pebbles rolling in a basin', showed an excess of *chi* in the body – possibly caused by a combination of the body's own *chi* and the presence of invading *chi* pouring in from outside (during pregnancy, when a

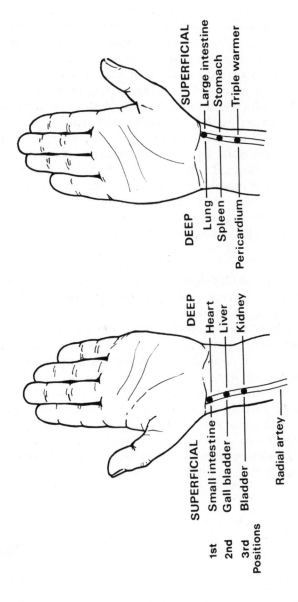

DEEP
Heart
Liver
Kidney

SUPERFICIAL
1st   Small intestine
2nd   Gall bladder
3rd   Bladder
Positions

Radial artey

SUPERFICIAL
Large intestine
Stomach
Triple warmer

DEEP
Lung
Spleen
Pericardium

Figure 14   *Positions of organs on the radial pulse.*

woman's *chi* was augmented by that of her child, this pulse was regarded as being normal); *hsien mo*, a taut pulse, felt as if the finger was pressed on a vibrating violin string, indicating that the liver may have been penetrated and damaged by the 'evil wind'; *huang mo*, a full, forceful, and bounding yang pulse, indicated an accumulation of heat, particularly in the triple warmer region; *sse mo* an intermittent pulse caused by a deficiency of blood and *chi*, indicated a deficiency in the yang organs, associated with a general malaise, chronic diarrhoea and coldness of the ears and nose; *k'ou mo*, a large, hollow, superficial, soft pulse (felt as if the finger was squeezing an onion stalk), followed a sudden loss of blood or dispersing of the yang constituent of *chi*; *hai mo*, a fine, soft, thread-like pulse, associated with a chronic debility and decaying *chi* content in the body; and *ch'ih mo*, a slow pulse (three beats to each breath), indicated the fact that cold had penetrated the yin interior.[6,7]

Those who are skilled at pulse diagnosis are really differentiating patients into relevant categories of traditional descriptions of disease. A modern physician in the Western world would separate patients into quite different descriptions of disease. It would be surprising indeed if the two assessments of a patient ever agreed; so it is pointless arguing for or against a diagnosis made in this way. One merely must record that this was the method employed by the traditional Chinese physicians – just as our methods today in the West will be regarded with some astonishment by our descendants.

Such diagnoses indicated by the pulse really make little sense in a modern setting, unless we really understand the various categories of disease that were described in ancient times.

5
Categories of Disease and the Planning of their Treatment

———————◆———————

The physician's attention was directed to the patient's whole state of health. Four pairs of principal entities or categories of disease had to be considered: 'external', 'internal'; 'cold' and 'hot'; 'deficiency' and 'excess'; 'yin' and 'yang'. Drs Lee and Cheung have recently published a splendid description of these complex categories of disease.[1]

External and internal
The patient's symptoms gave valuable clues as to whether the disease was 'external' or had progressed further *into* the body and had become 'internal' – thus affecting the viscera.

Take fever for example. If the disease was in its 'external' phase the symptoms and their causes were described as follows: a dread of cold; fever; headache; thin, pale, furry tongue; a floating pulse; etc.

Once the fever had become 'internal' the patient's symptoms and condition were considered to be far more serious: high fever; restlessness; mental dullness or delirium (indicating involvement of the heart); convulsions, or arching of the back so that only the head and heels rested on the bed (revealing an affected liver); abdominal pain and vomiting (associated with the stomach); shortness of breath, coughing and flaring of the nostrils (caused by the lungs); diarrhoea, dysentery or constipation (produced by malfunction of the spleen, large intestine and small intestine).

Hot and cold
The physician had to decide whether the predominant evils within a patient's body were of a 'hot' or 'cold' nature. An invasion of hot elements produced fever, thirst, a flushed face, a fully charged pulse, restlessness, dry stools, and a red tongue with yellow fur. 'Cold' elements, on the other hand, produced a pale face; a dread of the cold; cold limbs, a submerged, weak pulse, a desire to drink hot beverages; a low, feeble, mumbling voice; thin, loose stools, and a pale tongue with white fur.

Deficiency and excess
In 'deficiency' states the organs were thought to be depleted of their *chi*. 'Deficiency' illnesses were usually depressingly chronic in nature, causing the patient to develop a weak pulse and a low, nervous voice and to be unable to protrude his tongue vigorously. Often his face was withered.

In contrast, diseases of 'excess' were of short duration accompanied by a strong pulse, a flushed face, good spirits, loud voice and forceful protrusion of the tongue. Here there was an overabundance of *chi*: here the organs were imagined to be distended by the presence of two armies of *chi* battling for supremacy – the body's own *chi*, far from being depleted, being drawn up in full array for mortal combat with the 'evil' *chi* pouring in from outside.

Apparently 'deficiency' and 'excess' states sometimes co-existed in the same patient at the same time; for instance a fearful disease (which public health measures in the past two decades have virtually eradicated in China) called *schistoso-miasis*, contracted by working or bathing in contaminated water, was manifested by weakness and emaciation (or 'deficiency' disease) together with a grossly distended abdomen (signs of an 'excess' disease).

Yin and yang

Yin and yang elements pervaded all states of disease, whether they were 'internal' or 'external', 'cold' or 'hot', 'deficiency' or 'excessive'. Yin was associated with the 'internal', 'cold' and 'deficiency' states, while yang was associated with the 'external', 'hot' and 'excess' diseases.

It was not always as simple as that; various mixtures of diseases occurred – 'external cold', 'internal hot', 'deficiency hot' or 'excess cold'. In all of these it would have been difficult to decide whether yin or yang predominated. However, two conditions could be described without controversy: 'deficiency cold' had a classical yin description, while 'excess hot' was definitely a yang disease.

During the course of an illness the yin and yang elements often fluctuated. During an episode of pneumonia, for example, the patient normally began with yang manifestations: a flushed face, high fever, restlessness and a rapid strong pulse. Later the illness often progressed to a yin phase when the extremities became icy cold and the pulse became small and weak. A disease which passed from yang to yin in this way was regarded as being more likely to be mortal, while a disease which went from yin to yang was thought to be less dangerous. So every attempt was made to reverse the yin elements of a disease whenever possible. Warmth and hot drugs were used to try to draw the patient back from the fatal yin state.

Although each organ was by nature predominantly yin or yang, both elements were always present. Thus the heart, although a Lesser Yin organ, did contain yang elements in its *chi*, and a deficiency of these caused symptoms: shortness of breath; sweating at rest; coldness of the extremities, etc. These symptoms were quite different from those caused by a deficiency of the yin elements in the heart: palpitations; forgetfulness; sweating at night; and insomnia. Thus a careful history of the patient's symptoms gave some of the clues required to determine which elements had become depleted.

Planning the treatment of disease

If it was decided that any of the organs were filled to excess with *chi*, a particular manoeuvre was recommended to drain, calm or purge the excessive or 'evil' elements of *chi*. This manoeuvre was called 'sedation' or *xie*.

On the other hand, too empty an organ required another procedure called 'tonification' or *bu*; this was designed to supplement, fortify or stimulate the return of *chi* to the depleted organ; it also helped to drain off that which had become stagnant or unable to renew itself.[2]

Sedation

Vigorous manoeuvres were thought to be required to combat or disperse excessive or noxious elements of *chi* amassing in an organ.

The doctor and patient had to wait for a favourable moment: the day had to be warm with the moon in full phase; in all other respects the patient's body had to be in an orderly state.

Preferably a silver needle had to be thrust with a twisting movement rapidly into the meridian in the opposite direction to the flow of *chi* in the vessel. This procedure had to be carried out while the patient was breathing in.

Repeated entries into the blood stream were advised in the following manner: at every inhalation the needle-tip had to be advanced into the vessel and then partially withdrawn at every exhalation. In the meantime the needle was rotated anticlockwise in a rapid and energetic fashion.

Alternatively, another technique was often used – the 'push-and-pull' method. Here the needle was partially advanced and withdrawn rapidly; more force was used while pulling on the needle, literally with the idea of pulling yin out of the interior.

After the needle had been manipulated for approximately ten minutes, it was withdrawn slowly from the body, while the patient breathed out.[3,4]

Tonification

A milder technique was believed to be required for supplementing or *tonifying* organs depleted of *chi*. The needle was inserted at the end of exhalation to the required depth without rotation. The needle preferably was made of gold and inserted in the same direction as the flow of *chi* within the meridian. It was then twirled gently and slowly clockwise until the needle was 'gripped' by the tissue.

Again there was an alternative procedure – the 'push-and-pull' method. However on this occasion more force was employed in pushing the needle into the body than in pulling it back; this was designed to drive yang deep into the interior. The needle was withdrawn rapidly during inspiration while still being rotated clockwise. The 'hole' left by the needle insertion had to be massaged firmly by the physician's finger; this was called 'closing the hole'.

The entire procedure from start to finish occupied possibly half a minute.[4, 5]

6

The Five Laws of Acupuncture

———————◆———————

Once the student of traditional acupuncture had learnt the art of sedation and tonification, he was ready to consider the five laws of acupuncture, which were necessary to tell him what part of the patient's body required treatment.

A number of diagnostic observations were taken into account, quite apart from the taking of the pulses at the wrist. The colour of the complexion, the strength of the voice, the particular appearance of the tongue and the manner in which it was protruded, the appearance of the face and pupil of the eye were also considered together with a detailed history of the patient's condition. All of these and more were required to determine the state of all the organs.

One may readily imagine an almost infinite number of possible combinations of the states of each organ. For instance, a physician might decide a patient had too much *chi* in his liver, too little in his lungs and perhaps too much in his pericardium. Where then should he insert his needle and which manoeuvre should he perform?

There were five laws of acupuncture to guide him to the correct decision. Each one described a different set of rules that governed the interplay between the organs. The combination of all five laws gave the physician remarkable versatility in solving almost any problem.

It is worth describing these laws to reveal some of the intricate scholarship that must have been used in their design. It also shows that the physicians of those days had to think just as hard as their Western counterparts today – although of course the contents of their thoughts were quite different.

The names of the five laws were: (1) the law of five elements; (2) the circulation of *chi* with the pulses; (3) husband-and-wife; (4) midday, midnight; and (5) flow of *chi* through the meridians.

All of these were practised in China until the 1960s; since then the first of these – the law of five elements – appears to be the only one still being taught to beginners; perhaps the older generations of practitioners will be the only ones able to practise them all.

The law of the five elements

Between 350 and 270 BC, kings, dukes and powerful officials wooed the 'scientists' of their day. They even housed them in magnificent mansions with high gates and large halls in return for their scholarship and very practical advice in times of war.

The chief of these scientists, Master Tsou Yen, had kings sweeping the road for him as he passed on his way, and princes dusting his seat before he sat down. [1] He could look at his rulers with a level eye, for he knew the causes of natural events. He had studied China's great mountains, rivers and valleys, and knew the birds and beasts, the fruitfulness of China's waters and soils, and its rare products.

He spun a magnificent tapestry of ideas that explained all. His mastery of the yin and yang concepts explained cyclical events in history. He managed to combine nature's laws with politics and could explain the rise and fall of empires. He is credited with inventing or at least crystallising the theory of the five elements which were powerful forces flowing in a circle of wood, fire, earth, metal and water.

It is a remarkable fact that Tsou Yen's elder contemporary, Aristotle (384–322 BC), was laying down the seeds of European medicine by ascribing dry, hot, cold and moist qualities to the *four* elements known to the Greeks: earth, fire, air and water. Dr Joseph Needham compares the Greek and Chinese ideas about the elements, and notes that the Greeks did consider having a fifth element – aether – a subtler kind of air; but Aristotle felt that this was a substance of the heavenly bodies and not of this world.[2]

In the Chinese model the elements had a special relationship with each other; this followed the so-called 'father-and-son' law. Creative forces flowed from one element to another in the self-repeating cycle: wood, fire, earth, metal, water and wood, and so on.

> Heaven has five elements, first Wood, second Fire, third Earth, fourth Metal, and fifth Water. Wood comes first in the cycle of the five elements and water comes last, earth being in the middle. This is the order which Heaven has made. Wood produces fire, fire produces earth (i.e. ashes), earth produces metal (i.e. ores), metal produces water and water produces wood (for woody plants require water). This is their 'father-and-son' relation. . . . As transmitters they are fathers, as receivers they are sons. . . . Thus it is that the five elements correspond to the actions of filial sons and loyal ministers. Putting the five elements into words (like this) they really seem to be five kinds of action, do they not?[3]

This 'father-and-son' law was a vital concept to grasp. Take fire for example. Its 'father' was wood for two reasons: first of all twirling the fire-drill in various woods according to the season (elm and willow in the spring, jujube and apricot in the summer, oak and *yu* in autumn and *huai* and *than* in winter) kindled the fire,[4] while the wood itself fed the flames.

However, it was never to be forgotten that the activities of the 'son' appeared to have a reverse effect on the 'father'; for the simple act of fanning the flames of a fire tended to reduce the quantity of available wood. However, this same action produced more ashes which formed the substance of earth.

Thus, in Chinese medical terms, the act of tonifying fire sedated its 'father', wood; at the same time this action tonified its 'son', earth. On the other hand, sedating fire tonified wood and sedated earth.

Destructive cycle

Just as there was a creative cycle within the five elements there was also a destructive one.[5]

Wood, for example might give birth to fire; but it can also destroy earth (plants break up the soil and even crack rocks). The ashes from the fire may feed the earth; but fire melts metal. The ores from the earth provide metal; but earth may be used to build dykes to stop the progress of water. Metal when molten may resemble water (or water may be collected from dew that formed on metal mirrors that used to be left out at night for that purpose[6]); but metal cuts down wood. Water is required for the growth of wood; but water quenches fire.

Thus the destructive cycle ran through wood, earth, fire and metal to wood again. The 'father-and-son' law was applied to this cycle in reverse manner to the one that operated in the creative cycle.

The effects of this in studying the interactions of the elements in the destructive cycle were as follows: tonifying fire, for example, sedated its 'son', metal, and tonified its 'father', water; while sedating fire tonified metal and sedated water.

The two cycles combined

The two cycles may have been described (in Figure 15) as a pentagram of destruction contained within a circle of creation.

Flavour provides a link between the organs and the elements

Each element was associated with a flavour: water with saltiness (possibly because the naturalist scientists who concocted these ideas worked on the east coast and perhaps performed primitive experiments on crystallising salt from seawater); fire with bitterness (perhaps heat was used in the preparation of bitter medicines); wood with sourness (wood being vegetable was associated with many sour substances, particularly when decomposed); metal with acridity (this was probably associated with smelting procedures, which issued highly acrid fumes, for example sulphur dioxide); and earth with sweetness (bees' nests in the earth or the sweetness of various cereals).[7]

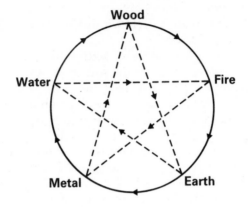

Continuous line – creative cycle.
Broken line – destructive cycle.

Figure 15   *The relationships of the five elements.*

It was perhaps but a step from giving flavours to the five elements to associating them with the various coupled organs of the body: gall bladder and liver were of the sour or 'wood' element; small intestine, heart, triple warmer and pericardium were gathered together around the bitter or 'fire' element; stomach and spleen were based in the sweet 'earth' element; large intestine and lung were accorded the acrid or pungent 'metal' element; while bladder and kidney were considered to be of the salty 'water' element.

In this way the yin and yang organs were evenly distributed amongst the elements.

Operating the law of five elements

In this law, however, the activity of yin organs was thought only to affect other yin organs; while yang organs were supposed to act exclusively on yang organs. Thus, to understand the system, two separate diagrams were required, one for the yin organs and another for the yang organs (see Figure 16).

The 'father-and-son' law was thought to operate both through the destructive and creative cycles: for example,

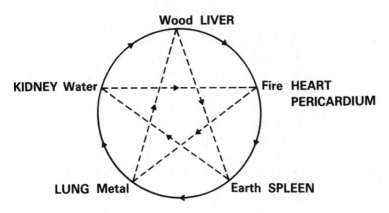

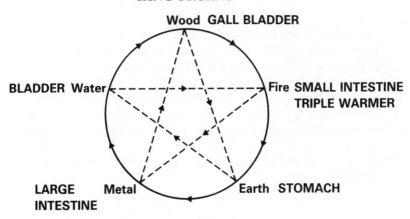

Continuous line – creative cycle.
Broken line – destructive cycle.

Figure 16   *The law of five elements applied to yin and yang organs.*

the act of tonifying the 'wood' organ, the liver (see the upper of the two diagrams in Figure 16), was believed to have various effects on all the other yin organs: (i) on the *creative cycle* (outer circle) according to the father-and-son law, the 'water' organ, the kidney, would have been sedated, while the 'fire' organs, the heart and pericardium, were being tonified; (ii) according to the *destructive* cycle (dotted lines) where the father-and-son law operated in reverse, the 'earth' organ, the spleen, would have been sedated, while the 'metal' organ, the lung, was tonified.

Once the physician had diagnosed the irregular nature of his patient's flow of *chi*, and determined the most effective method of restoring order, he still had to decide where the needles should be inserted to carry out the required sedation or tonification. This difficulty is described in more detail in the next chapter.

However that was not the end of the matter: there were the four other laws to consider as well; these had to be applied at the same time.

Four other laws of acupuncture

The four other laws were: The circulation of *chi* through the pulses; husband-and-wife; midday midnight; and flow of *chi* through the meridians. The first two laws behaved in a similar way to the law of five elements limiting the influence of yin to yin organs and of yang to yang organs; whilst the last two allowed the activities of yin organs to affect yang organs and vice versa. Dr Felix Mann translated and described them lucidly in his book *Acupuncture: The Ancient Chinese Art of Healing*.[8]

Circulation of *chi* through the pulses

To operate this law, the position of each organ's influence on the radial pulse had to be studied (see Figure 14, page 57). As in the law of five elements, the yin organs were separated from the yang.

The flow of *chi* through the yin occurred in the following cycle (see Table 4): heart, pericardium, spleen, lung, kidney, liver and round to heart again. Tonification of one of these organs had the effect of tonifying the organ immediately before or after it. (Thus tonifying the lung, for example, also tonified the spleen and kidneys.)

The same rule applied to the yang organs, whose separate cycle was: small intestine, 'triple warmer', stomach, large intestine, bladder, gall bladder and back to small intestine again. Thus, tonifying triple warmer tonified the small intestine and stomach.

Table 4   *Circulation of* chi *through the pulses*

Positions on the radial pulse			Radial pulses		
			Left		*Right*
YIN ORGANS	Deep	First	HEART		LUNG
	Deep	Second	LIVER		SPLEEN
	Deep	Third	KIDNEY		PERI-CARDIUM
YANG ORGANS	Super-ficial	First	SMALL INTESTINE		LARGE INTESTINE
	Super-ficial	Second	GALL BLADDER		STOMACH
	Super-ficial	Third	BLADDER		TRIPLE WARMER

Husband-and-wife law

This law also required the knowledge of the positions on the radial pulse (see Figure 14, page 57).

Again the yin and yang organs were separated (see Table 5).

On this occasion tonification of an organ was only successful if the organ in the same position but on the opposite pulse had a surplus of *chi* to transfer to it. Thus if the large intestine was depleted of *chi*, and the small intestine had too much, then tonifying the large intestine corrected the balance.

Table 5   *Husband-and-wife law*

Positions on the radial pulse			Radial pulses		
			Left		*Right*
YIN ORGANS	Deep	First	HEART	⟷	LUNG
	Deep	Second	LIVER	⟷	SPLEEN
	Deep	Third	KIDNEY	⟷	PERI-CARDIUM
YANG ORGANS	Super-ficial	First	SMALL INTESTINE	⟷	LARGE INTESTINE
	Super-ficial	Second	GALL BLADDER	⟷	STOMACH
	Super-ficial	Third	BLADDER	⟷	TRIPLE WARMER

Midday-midnight law

Chi flowed through the various organs in a regular sequence. Each organ tended to reach a peak of activity at different times of the day, shown in Table 6.

A wonderful but complicated passage from the *Classic of Internal Medicine* describes the influence of time on the various categories of yin and yang:

> It is said that there is Yin within Yin and that there is Yang within Yang. Thus from early dawn until midday there prevails the Yang of Heaven which is Yang within the Yang. From midday until twilight there prevails the Yang of Heaven which is the Yin within the Yang. From the time when night encloses the Earth until the first crowing of the cock there prevails the Yin of Heaven which is the Yin within the Yin. From the cock's crowing until early morning there prevails the Yin of Heaven which is the Yang within the Yin.[9]

The importance of the midday-midnight law lay in the fact that it provided a mechanism for yin organs to affect yang organs, and vice versa.

Again the arrangement of the organs at the radial pulse (Figure 14, p. 57) had an influence. On this occasion the coupled organs that occupied positions on the left radial pulse were arranged in yin and yang columns above those that had an influence on the right radial pulse.

This arrangement reveals pairs of organs that were believed to reach peak activities at opposite times of day. In Table 6 organs in each pair that behaved in this way are linked by arrows; it will be seen that the heart, for example, was thought to be most active at midday, while its opposite fellow, the gall bladder waited until midnight.

Each pair of organs were thought to be linked by a secondary meridian in such a way that if an organ was strongly tonified it would attract surplus *chi* (provided that it was present) from its opposite number.

Table 6   *Midday-midnight law*

Radial pulses	Time of peak activity	Yin		Yang	Time of peak activity
LEFT WRIST	midday	HEART	✕	SMALL INTESTINE	2 p.m.
	2 a.m.	LIVER		GALL BLADDER	midnight
	6 p.m.	KIDNEY	✕	BLADDER	4 p.m.
RIGHT WRIST	4 a.m.	LUNG		LARGE INTESTINE	6 a.m.
	10 a.m.	SPLEEN	✕	STOMACH	8 a.m.
	8 p.m.	PERI- CARDIUM		TRIPLE WARMER	10 p.m.

Flow of *chi* through the meridians

Chi flowed through the twelve main meridians in a continuous circle (see Figure 6, page 35); in fact *chi* was supposed to leap from an 'exit' point on one main meridian and to pass down a connecting vessel to an 'entry' point in the next main meridian in the cycle.

The 'exit' points were usually located near the end of one meridian where it passed close to the 'entry' point of the next. The favourite places for meridians to meet lay in the hand, shoulder region of the chest, head and foot.

The law of the flow of *chi* through the meridians stated that if a point of 'entry' was tonified, tonification was only successful if the previous meridian had excess *chi* to pass on to it; the effect of this exercise also sedated the previous meridian's organ.

If a point of 'exit' was sedated, sedation only occurred if the next meridian was deficient in *chi* and allowed the excess to be passed on to it; the result therefore tonified the next meridian's organ.

This law had the advantage that treatment of a yang organ affected the state of a yin organ, and vice versa.

7
The Acupuncture Points

◆

The main meridians provided the physician with a means of effecting the required sedation or tonification.

Each organ's main meridian had close communication with the skin at various sites called 'acupuncture points'. These points acted as pores which were able to open or close; they allowed external events to influence the flow of *chi* within the meridians. They also allowed internal secretions to escape, weakening the body: 'When the body uses all its strength, perspiration flows freely through the open pores and encounters the minute but weakening influences within man.'[1] Yet at the same time the escape of perspiration through the 'pores' served as a natural relief of excessive *chi*: 'The perspiration which is generated by Yang is of the same importance as the rain, which is generated by the Universe.'[2]

The physician was able to insert needles into these pores or acupuncture points and, depending on his method, effect profound changes in the flow of *chi* within the meridian which in turn affected the organs themselves.

The five laws of acupuncture worked to allow the physician the opportunity of *redressing the balance* when various combinations of organs were disturbed either by an excess or deficiency of *chi*. To achieve this each main meridian had five important acupuncture points – 'father', 'own', 'son', 'entry' and 'exit' points.

'Father', 'own' and 'son' points

Each main meridian had wood, fire, earth, metal and water points at various sites below the elbows or knees, as the case may be (see Figures 17 and 18).

Its 'own' point was the one belonging to its own element. Thus the water point was the kidney's 'own' point, as the kidney was a water organ.

The kidney's 'father' point was its metal point as, according to the law of the five elements, metal gave birth to water.

The same law was used to show that the 'son' point of the kidney was its wood point, for water nourishes wood.

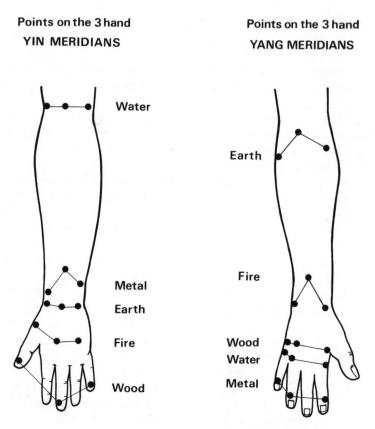

Points on the 3 hand
YIN MERIDIANS

Water

Metal
Earth

Fire

Wood

Points on the 3 hand
YANG MERIDIANS

Earth

Fire

Wood
Water

Metal

Figure 17   *Important points on the meridians on the upper limb.*

Tonification of 'own' point

The law of five elements explained when to tonify an organ's 'own' point: when its son was deficient and its mother was overburdened with *chi* on its creative cycle, and its opposing organ on the destructive cycle was overabundant – then tonifying its 'own' point corrected the matter. (If the opposing organ on its destructive cycle was depleted of *chi*, then sedating the meridian's 'own' point restored the balance.)

The same law was used to show how an organ suffering from excess was sedated by tonifying its 'son' point.

The law of circulation of *chi* through the pulses revealed

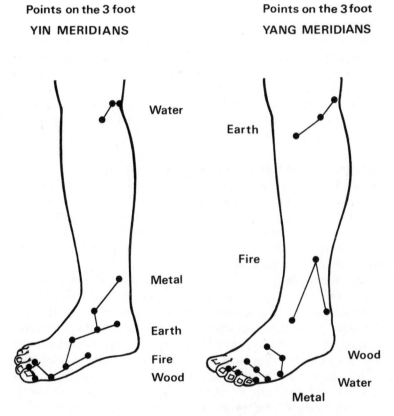

Points on the 3 foot

YIN MERIDIANS

Points on the 3 foot

YANG MERIDIANS

Water

Earth

Fire

Metal

Earth

Fire

Wood

Wood

Water

Metal

Figure 18   *Important points on the meridians on the lower limb.*

other phenomena: tonification of an organ's 'own' point restored deficient organs lying in positions before and after it (see Table 4, page 71).

Meanwhile the law of husband-and-wife indicated yet other possibilities: if an organ was depleted of *chi*, and the organ represented in the same position on the opposite pulse happened to have an excess, then tonification of the deficient organ's 'own' point would allow the excess to be transmitted to it (see Table 5, page 72).

The midday-midnight law showed how strong tonification of an empty organ's 'own' point removed any excess from the organ whose activities reached a maximum at the opposite time of day (see Table 6, page 73).

Entry and exit points

The law of the flow of *chi* through the meridians demonstrated that when an organ was low in *chi*, while its preceding organ was too full – then tonifying its 'entry' point rectified the problem.

On the other hand if an organ was bursting with excessive *chi*, and its successor was empty – then sedating its 'exit' point restored normality.

Integration of the five laws of acupuncture

Remarkably few contradictions appear when all five laws are studied together; for they were the work of considerable scholarship and were all designed to augment each other. Perhaps a description of the various combinations that could be treated by one point at a time on the lung main meridian may serve as an example:

When the lung, spleen and kidneys were deficient at the same time as an excess appeared in the heart, bladder and liver, tonification of but one point, the lung's 'mother point', was the only procedure required. When the kidney was deficient, and the spleen and liver carried excess *chi*, then tonification of the lung's 'own point' was the correct treatment; sedating this point, however, was mandatory when only the liver was deficient. If the lung alone was supporting an excess of *chi*, then the lung's 'son' point had to be tonified; on the other hand if the lung was the only organ to be deficient, then tonifying the lung's 'entry' point was the correct procedure. Meanwhile, tonifying the lung's 'exit' point was required when an excess appeared in the lung and a deficiency of *chi* was manifest in the large intestine.

Acupuncture point classification

Although only six points on each of the twelve main meridians represented on both sides of the body have been described so far, there were many others – making a total of 309. These were divided amongst the meridians in the following way:

meridians	number of points
lung	11
large intestine	20
stomach	45
spleen	21
heart	9
small intestine	19
bladder	67
kidney	27
pericardium	9
triple warmer	23
gall bladder	44
liver	14

Fifty-two other points lay on the mid-line of the trunk and head (twenty-four on the Conception Vessel and twenty-eight on the Governing Vessel) making a grand total of 361.[3]

The Yellow Emperor, however, arrived at a different total: 'Following the course of each of the arteries there are the (365) vital points for acupuncture. Each of these points has a place and a name. . . .'[4]

The names of the points had meanings that were sometimes mysterious and beautiful. For example, translations of some of the Conception Vessel points reveal this: Jade Court (*Yutang*); Heaven Rushing Out (*Tiantu*); Flower Covering (*Huagai*); Dove Tail (*Jiuwei*); and Middle Hall (*Zhongting*).

Often the particular meanings of the points helped the student to remember their functions; for instance, Leg Three Miles (*Zusanli*), a point on the stomach meridian, indicated that part of the leg just below the knee (on the outer aspect) which frequently begins to hurt after walking some distance. Treatment of this point tended to increase the distance the patient could walk without pain. A region near the nose (*Yingxiang*) was called the point of Welcome Fragrance as treatment of this improved the patient's sense of smell.

The distribution of acupuncture points

The 361 named acupuncture points were distributed in the body in the following way: 75 were to be found in the head region; 63 lay on each arm; 139 were to be found on the trunk; and 84 were located on each leg.

In addition, there were 36 extra points described on either side of the body which did not lie on any of the meridians. Each of these had its own specific functions.

In fact, the number of extra points has been steadily growing and a book has been published with the splendid title, *Points: 2001*.[5]

Approximately 80 per cent of the 361 acupuncture points lay over muscles; with very few exceptions these points lay at either end of muscles or along their free borders. The remainder (20 per cent) lay directly over bony structures such as the vertebrae or fingers and toes. (In fact, only 18 out of the 83 most commonly used points recently selected by the Peking Academy of Traditional Chinese Medicine[6] lie over bony points.)

Numbered points

The French, who have been practising acupuncture for at least 300 years, preferred to describe acupuncture points numerically.

The direction of the flow of *chi* down the meridian would be taken into account; for instance, the pericardium meridian arises in the chest and flows down the arm towards the middle finger. The first point in the chest would be titled 'Pericardium 1'; as there were only nine points in this meridian, the last point on the tip of the middle finger was called 'Pericardium 9'.[7]

This had the advantage that, as long as the direction of the meridian was known, any point described in this way could be found rapidly from an atlas. In recent years the Chinese themselves have introduced a similar numbering system; unfortunately the numbers they have chosen are not identical in all instances.

Classes of acupuncture points

Various acupuncture points were classed together as they shared similar effects on the body when stimulated. One of the most interesting groups were the *Bei-Shu* points. These were arranged on the back at either side of the spine from the middle of the chest downwards. They were reputed to become reflexly tender when various organs were diseased.

These points referred to the organs from above downwards in the following way: lung; pericardium; heart; liver; gall bladder; spleen; stomach; triple warmer; kidney; large intestine; small intestine; and bladder. Thus, once this system was known, discovering the precise location of a tender area in the back helped practitioners to diagnose which organ was diseased; furthermore, stimulating a *Bei-Shu* point was believed to assist a damaged organ's function. These *Bei-Shu* points were based on astute observations; for they heralded similar Western medical studies which confirm them in a general way.

Similarly, on the front of the chest and abdomen, other points called Alarm or *Mo* points were described. Again, these were reflexly tender and indicated the condition of various organs. These points were scattered down the sides of the body and also in the mid-line.

Other categories of points, more difficult to grasp by the Western-trained doctor, included such ideas as the 'meeting points'; these occurred apparently where one or more meridians crossed over each other. Needling a 'meeting point' was thought to affect the meridians linked in this way.

Approximately 70 per cent of the 361 acupuncture points had some other function besides its own – it might be a wood, fire, water, meeting, *Bei-Shu*, *Mo*, source, exit point, and so on.

Location of acupuncture points

Students were taught how to locate acupuncture points as accurately as possible. Although carefully produced statues and atlases of the human form were produced, these were not ideal as patients came in all shapes and sizes.

To overcome the disparity between the shape of a particular patient and the atlas portraying an average body, a surprisingly ingenuous unit of measure was introduced – the Chinese inch (variously spoken of as a *cun* or *tsun*). The idea behind this was that if a patient was uncommonly tall he would be expected to have long fingers. The Chinese inch was taken to be the length of the middle bone in his middle finger – see Figure 22, page 145. A special protractor has been designed to measure the length of this bone in any patient and this can be used to discover the location of the various points; for each point is defined as being so many Chinese inches away from the various bony landmarks on the body.

Each point was thought of as existing at a certain depth below the skin. This too was measured in Chinese inches, and to reach a certain point the needle had to be inserted to the prescribed depth. Thus a mastery of acupuncture required a very detailed study of the surface anatomy of the body and an appreciation of the structures that lay at various depths beneath the skin; for some points were thought of as being as much as three Chinese inches below the skin.

Forbidden points

Drs Anton Jayasuriya and Felix Fernando have written an interesting section on the 'forbidden' points or those points which should never be needled in their book *Principles and Practice of Scientific Acupuncture*, published in Sri Lanka.[8] They mention the fact that in the ancient sources twenty-eight forbidden points were listed. They have succeeded in narrowing the list to ten. These are forbidden for obvious anatomical reasons. The first acupuncture point on the stomach meridian, for instance, lies in the orbital cavity containing the eyeball; a needle placed here might well endanger a patient's eye. Other points lie in the neck directly over the carotid arteries or the trachea (windpipe). Many points on the chest which were not specifically listed in this description of forbidden points lie directly over the lung; penetration of the lung with an acupuncture needle may cause pneumothorax (rupture of the lung), which might be fatal if not treated.

However, a patient seeking the attention of a practitioner who has gained his knowledge of anatomy at a medical school and has kept himself up to date on this subject would be at little risk, for these practitioners assiduously avoid dangerous locations.

8
Instruments of Acupuncture and Moxibustion

◆

A whole host of fascinating techniques were employed in the practice of acupuncture and 'moxibustion', or the administration of heat.

Acupuncture needles
Drs Alan Klide and Shiu Kung, who are interested in the veterinary use of acupuncture in the United States, give an excellent description of the nine types of needle that have been employed:[1]

1   The chisel needle, whose blade was shaped like an arrowhead, was used in treating skin diseases.
2   The round needle had an egg-shaped tip and was used for massage.
3   The spoon needle had a round blade, which was used for pressing on the skin.
4   The lance needle had a prism-like blade sharp on three sides; this was used for blood-letting.
5   The stiletto needle was curved like a sword for draining.
6   The round, sharp needle was used to relieve pain by being quickly inserted and strongly stimulated.
7   The long needle was used in areas of thick fascia and muscle. Sometimes these needles reached three feet in length.

8   The big needle was principally used in a form of treatment
    called moxibustion where the actual shaft of the needle
    was heated to a high temperature by burning specially pre-
    pared herbs wrapped round its handle.
9   The soft hair needle is the one usually used today (see
    Figure 1, page 5) and as its name implies has an extremely
    thin diameter.

All of these needles were described by the Yellow Emperor
as if they were made of iron; but there has been considerable
controversy about other metals being employed. Drs Chimin
Wong and Leinteh Wu described these in their *History of
Chinese Medicine*.[2] According to them the yellow metals (gold
and copper) had a yang or stimulating, vivifying power, while
the white metals (silver, chrome and zinc) had a yin or calm-
ing, dispersing power.

In the tenth century AD mild (low-carbon) steel used for
making horses' bits was considered the best substance to make
needles from; the ancients named needles constructed from
such steel *chin chen* to indicate their value as tough yet
malleable instruments. This title has been misinterpreted to
mean that they were made of gold.[3] Nevertheless, both silver
and gold, if they were employed, have antiseptic qualities;
perhaps less infection occurred with their use. Precious metals
would have had the added advantage of not becoming
corroded with rust.

Grey metals (iron, steel, platinum, etc.) were regarded by
the purists as being neutral metals.[4] Certainly, the shafts of
most modern acupuncture needles are made of stainless steel.

Other types of acupuncture instruments
Porcelain needles are still used today in the Kwangsi province
of China; they were originally made of Pien stone. Drs Lee
and Cheung describe how people there lightly knock pieces of
broken porcelain or china with the back of a knife to make
sharp porcelain chips. They place them in boiling water for
half an hour to partially sterilise them.[5]

A modern version of the round needle originally described
by the Yellow Emperor is the 'push' needle. This is about four
inches long and made out of thick steel wire or hard wood.

The needle-tip is too blunt to pierce the skin. Scraping the tip over the skin and pushing or pressing it at the same time can produce the required result.

Another instrument is shaped like a hammer. The head of the hammer contains a cluster of fine needles; repeated hammering with this instrument using the appropriate amount of pressure along the course of the meridian can be employed. This type of instrument has also been used with children as it is relatively painless and swift in its application.

To cover a wider area, an instrument shaped like a garden roller with needles sticking out of its surface has been used.

Sometimes special instruments called *trocar* and *cannula* are employed. A plastic tube (or *cannula*) with holes in it, kept temporarily rigid by an internal needle (or *trocar*), is driven through the skin. The needle is removed and solutions of various kinds can be introduced into the *cannula* which is now lying under the skin. Such solutions may be normal saline, 10 per cent glucose solutions, distilled water, vitamin B_1, vitamin B_{12}, local anaesthetic, and various types of herbal extracts.

Strong forms of treatment

More drastic techniques have been developed which sometimes do not use needles at all; many of these are used today. Incisions, for example, may be made in the skin and the fatty tissue from the wound excised. On other occasions the needle is inserted through the skin and twisted so that the fibrous elements in the skin grip the needle, the needle is then removed from the skin with the fibrous tissue still sticking to it; these threads of fibrous tissue are then severed.

Suture material (catgut) is sometimes inserted via a hollow lumbar puncture needle and buried under the skin, usually within muscles. The length of the suture material may be arranged in a figure of eight to cover a wide area. The suture material excites various reactions within the body and is slowly absorbed.

Specific nerve trunks may be dissected and electrically stimulated.

An ancient form of strong treatment applied to large areas of the skin was called 'cupping'. This was also used in the

West and is still used in China. Here a vessel made of metal, bamboo or glass is heated up and placed over the skin. When it cools, a vacuum is formed causing a bruise the size of the orifice of the vessel.

Relatively painless treatment

Most readers who might be considering having acupuncture will probably close the book at this stage and seek help elsewhere. However it must be remembered that the Chinese physicians of bygone times were faced with all manner of diseases and had no modern antibiotics, anaesthetics or surgery.

Severe illnesses required heroic remedies. Fortunately the medically qualified acupuncturist of today is merely using this treatment as an adjunct to all the other methods at his disposal. Today great efforts are made to use the *least* painful stimulus required to achieve the desired effect; often patients are unaware that any needles have been inserted at all.

Nevertheless, it is worth recording these traditional practices as they give valuable clues to acupuncture's possible mechanisms of action.

Moxibustion

Moxibustion is a form of therapy where heat is applied either to the needle or to the skin. The Chinese developed a remarkably ingenious use of natural resources employing a specially prepared herb of the *Artemisia* genus. Between March and May of each year thick leaves were collected, dried under sunlight and then ground into fine fragments with a mortar and pestle.[6] Any impurities such as soil or sand were strained off and the whole process was repeated until a fine, clean, white, soft, textured 'wool' held together by its fibres was obtained. This was called moxa wool and its fineness depended on the number of times this refining procedure had been carried out. Moxa wool had the advantage that when rolled up in the shape of a cigar and lit at one end it would burn steadily, transmitting an even heat.

Portions of the fine moxa wool could be moulded around the handle of a needle and ignited. A rather thicker needle was used for this purpose so that the heat was transmitted from the handle to the tissues of the body where the shaft of the needle lay.

Small cones of moxa were placed directly on the skin itself and the tip of the cone was lit (coarse moxa wool sufficed for this purpose).

The fiery nature of this treatment revealed its yang qualities. Its use was recommended by the *Classic of Internal Medicine*:

> The (evil) winds contribute to the development of a hundred diseases. When the present wind is cold and it strikes man, it will cause his body hair to stand out straight and it will cause his skin to be stopped up, and man will become hot and feverish. At that time he can perspire and thus send forth (the evil influences within). But it is also possible that numbness brings about swellings and pains. At that time one must apply hot liquids and hot irons and finally resort to fire which is used in burning moxa for cauterisation and thus bring about the disappearance (of the evil winds).[7]

Direct moxibustion could be augmented by mixing in aromatic powders (*Flos caryophylli* and *Cortex cinnamoni*) which facilitated the amount of heat production.

Garlic juice could be smeared over the skin at the desired place so that the moxa cone would stick closely to it. In addition, garlic has its own irritative qualities to the skin.

When the heat from the moxa became extremely painful, the physician massaged the skin around the cone to alleviate the burning pain. When the cone had burnt itself out, the skin was bathed in water. This process was repeated sometimes up to nine times. The result of this formed a burn which often took thirty or forty days to heal. These burns frequently became infected.

Those physicians who still use moxibustion prefer to use the 'indirect method'; this reduces the risk of burning the patient by interposing a piece of garlic or ginger between the cone and the skin. When the heat becomes painful the moxa cone is immediately removed and the skin is allowed to cool.

A remarkable number of methods and substances have been

used for moxibustion. When treating carbuncles and boils, for instance, yellow earth and water was mixed to a muddy consistency, and rolled into a cake. This cake was placed over the carbuncle and a burning pinch of moxa was placed on top of that. Another method was to make a circle of wet flour around the base of the carbuncle; melted beeswax was poured onto the carbuncle layer by layer. As each layer hardened and cooled another warm layer would be added. Another method would be to roll the moxa into a form of a tube or cigar and set fire to it at one end. This could be applied directly to the handle of the needle or to the skin.

The difference between acupuncture and moxibustion
Using an acupuncture needle on its own was regarded as being a yin form of treatment, while moxibustion was definitely a yang form of therapy. Indeed, the difference between the two forms of treatment was heightened by the existence of a special chart showing only thirty-three points which should be used for moxibustion.[8]

The clever physician was able to determine the yin and yang qualities of his patient and hence the indication for either acupuncture or moxibustion by studying his patient's (yin) pulse and (yang) complexion very carefully: the yang component of *chi* lay outside meridians and protected the flesh itself – thus contributing to the complexion; the yin component was judged on the quality of the pulses: 'the complexion corresponds to the sun, the pulse corresponds to the moon. If one is constant in one's search for their meaning one will discover the importance of the complexion and the pulse.'[9]

9
The Superior Physician in Ancient China

◆

There was an idea that the physician could monitor the yin and yang influences on the body and detect any alterations in their natural harmony at a very early stage of disease. This had important implications: the superior physician could keep a watch over any evil influences before they had time to develop and damage the patient's health permanently; while the inferior physician had to wait until the disease manifested itself before he could treat the patient, when perhaps it was already too late.

> The superior physician helps before the early budding of disease. He must first examine the three regions of the body and define the atmosphere of the nine subdivisions so that they are entirely in harmony, and nothing can be destroyed, and then his help sets in. Therefore he is called the superior physician.
>
> The inferior physician begins to help when (the disease) has already developed; he helps when destruction has already set in. And since his help comes when the disease has already developed it is said of him that he is ignorant.[1]

The dangers of being a superior physician
However, it was at times dangerous to be too 'superior' a

physician. In the second century AD there was supposed to be a remarkable doctor called Hua Tho.

He even dared to perform certain surgical procedures. He carried out amputations, reunited severed limbs, and even removed diseased parts of bowel – sewing together the healthy portion and spreading a whitish powder over the wounds to prevent infection. (Perhaps he had also discovered a penicillin-like substance.)

He anaesthetised his patients with a 'dream medicine'[2] (*ma fei san* – a mixture of hemp and wine). However, he was selective in its use, and refused to use *ma fei san* in obstetric emergencies as he recognised its dangers for mother and baby; on these occasions he used acupuncture instead.

His prowess led him to his execution at the hands of the war lords.

It all began when he treated a great warrior Kuan Yu, who had been hit in the arm by a poisoned arrow while battling with the Lord of Northern China, Tshao Tshao. During the operation Kuan Yu spurned the 'dream medicine' as he was anxious to keep his wits about him. While Hua Tho opened his arm and scraped the bone, he continued to play *Go* (a Chinese form of chess) – see Plate 7.

Tshao Tshao was amazed to see Kuan Yu return fresh to the fray after what should have been a fatal wound; he was determined to learn the name of the excellent physician.

At a later date Tshao Tshao gradually became plagued by severe headaches. Unannounced he called upon Hua Tho and sought his advice. Hua Tho diagnosed a brain tumour, which he offered to remove surgically. Tshao Tshao suspected that this was an attempt to assassinate him and commanded Hua Tho to find some other way to relieve his headaches.

Tshao Tshao's symptoms included headaches, mental disturbance and dizziness; all of these were treated successfully by Hua Tho, who decided to needle one point on the sole of the foot.

Apparently Hua Tho was very sparing with the use of his needles and particularly asked his patient to report any sensations he received during treatment. This description almost certainly tells us that *techi* (the unpleasant or bizarre sensations deliberately sought by deep needling (see page 144) already formed an important part of acupuncture even at so early a date as the second century AD).[3]

Tshao Tshao was so impressed that he abducted Hua Tho to treat the rest of his followers. As the mighty doctor's sympathies lay with Kuan Yu, he made every effort to escape. On one of these occasions he was recaptured and executed. Not long afterwards, Tshao Tshao died of the brain tumour that Hua Tho had diagnosed.

While lying in prison Hua Tho was unable to tell his wife how important his papers were; she used them to light her kitchen stove. Nevertheless, apparently a few of his works have survived, including some anatomical descriptions gained from his surgical experiences.

However a Chinese historian Ch'en Heng-ch'ueh dismissed these stories as a Chinese version of a Buddhist religious myth from India.[4] In any event surgery ceased in China from that time onwards until the present century.

Hua Tho's story tells us that acupuncture was just one of several methods of treating disease. The Chinese were never afraid to explore herbal remedies, diets, advice on behaviour, exercises, manipulation, and massage, as well as the use of the needle and heat to assuage man's ills.

However there still remains the question: Which elements of acupuncture's practice, if any, deserve to be investigated in a modern scientific manner? Perhaps we ought to see how modern medicine was developed and therefore how today's doctors use their knowledge to test the traditional Chinese claims; for if any of these pass the test they will form part of the full armament of modern medicine.

Part Three

Modern Acupuncture

In 1958 the Chinese discovered that patients could undergo major surgery in relative comfort under the influence of acupuncture instead of a general anaesthetic. 80,000 operations were carried out in this way by 1973.[1] Although as we will see the success of this technique was probably exaggerated at first, it has given Western-trained doctors the necessary impetus to study acupuncture in a scientific manner.

Both Chinese and Western laboratories have shown that patients respond to the needles by producing their own form of morphine. This work will be described in greater detail in Chapter 12; it gave the Chinese the opportunity to start to integrate their traditional methods of medicine with Western developments. As a result, it will be surprising indeed if many of acupuncture's mechanisms are not better understood in the near future.

However, Western practitioners who slavishly follow what they think is the traditional system of acupuncture may not welcome the attention of scientists. Their fear would be that once their methods were 'investigated' the most effective elements would be improved while the nonsensical ones would be thrown away. They might well demand, 'What right have scientists to tamper with so complete and scholarly a system of medicine that has persisted so long and given so much comfort to millions of people?'

Scientists do carry awesome responsibilities to truth. Huxley described the great tragedy of science as 'the slaying of a beautiful hypothesis by an ugly fact'.[2] He also described the scientist's methods: 'Science is nothing but trained and organised common sense, differing from the latter only as veteran may differ from a raw recruit: and its methods differ from those of common sense only as far as the guardsman's cut and thrust differ from the manner in which a savage wields his club'.[3]

Some clever practitioners have adapted well to this threat and pretend to be as scientific as possible to blind and bind patients to their practice:

> Of science and logic he chatters
>   As fine and as fast as he can;
> Though I am no judge of such matters,
>   I am sure he is a talented man.
> > Winthrop Mackworth Praed
> > (1802–39), 'The Talented Man'

Yet others like to take a global approach to their task and talk loftily in vague generalities about treating the 'whole body' and so forth. The poets had something to say about them too:

> He who would do good to another must do it in
>   Minute Particulars.
>
> General Good is the plea of the scoundrel, hypocrite,
>   and flatterer;
>
> For Art and Science cannot exist but in minutely
>   organized Particulars.
> > William Blake (1757–1827), 'Jerusalem'

It is difficult to define scientific methods: perhaps a more honest description is that science is nothing more than a consensus amongst scientists. Naturally this evolves at much the same speed as any other shared view of the world. One should never hold the priggish view that scientists are always right. Most original thinkers bubble over with ideas; it is all too easy to be convinced of the 'truth' of one's own ideas and not look hard enough at possible criticisms. Lord Russell Brain, a distinguished British neurologist, wrote: 'The progress of science depends upon the ability to ride with one foot on each of two horses, one named Fact and the other Hypothesis, and the problem is to keep them running level.'[4]

We are all forced to specialise, as the days of universal learning are over. The amount of scientific literature on the subject of acupuncture alone written in the past three decades has exceeded anything written on the subject by the Chinese before that date.

My hope is that this section will give the reader an introduction to these new developments and perhaps illustrate how the West has not turned her back on valuable ideas from China. Indeed, there are signs that the Chinese experience will steadily evolve under Western-inspired scrutiny into a really worthwhile method of relief for many of man's ills.

10

The Birth of Modern Medicine

---◆---

Modern medicine was probably born in the 1830s in Europe; about that time doctors began to question the whole ritual of medicine, which then included cupping, purging, bleeding, diets of every conceivable sort and the use of a wide variety of plant extracts. They began to ask the question whether these 'remedies' actually harmed the patient and prolonged his illness.

With courage and considerable self-restraint many doctors decided to watch and wait, giving only sensible advice – advocating bed-rest, nourishing diets, good nursing routines and other purely supportive measures. For the first and possibly last time, they took the opportunity to witness the natural history of untreated disease.

Patients were not always impressed by this approach:

> Nor bring, to see me cease to live,
> Some doctor full of phrase and fame,
> To shake his sapient head and give
> The ill he cannot cure a name!
>
> Matthew Arnold, 'A Wish'

The doctor's chief and apparently inactive role was to explain to the patient's family the likely course of events and allay any needless anxieties. This allowed him to study his patients with painstaking care, recording every step of their illnesses. He took to heart Hippocrates' maxim:

> Consider what has gone before, recognize the signs before your eyes and then make your progress. Practise two things in your dealings with disease; either help or do not harm the patient. There are three factors in the practice of medicine: the disease, the patient and the physician. The physician is the servant of science, and the patient must do what he can to fight the disease with the assistance of the physician. [1]

These profound words, probably written during the fifth century BC, were appreciated by the austere Victorians in their approach to medicine. It was not long before many diseases could be separated from each other by reading the records of their history; for the first time, for instance, typhus and typhoid were shown to be quite different diseases.

Circulation of blood: theories in China and the West

Meanwhile fundamental changes were taking place in the understanding of how the body functions.

We are indebted to Drs Joseph Needham and Lu Gwei-Djen for pointing out in their valuable work *Celestial Lancets*[2] that the Chinese had already described the circulation of blood in ancient texts:[3] 'What we call the vascular system (Mo) is like dykes and retaining walls (forming a circular tunnel) which control the path which is traversed by the Yin Chi so that it can not escape or anywhere leak away.' A Ming-dynasty commentary (written no later than AD 1586) throws even more light on the circulation: 'It means that Yin Chi travels within blood vessels round and round, day and night, meeting nothing to stop or oppose it, and that is what the blood vessels are.'

The idea that blood flowed in a continuous circulation through the organs was far from clear in the West.

Aristotle (384–322 BC) taught that blood was formed in the liver and was distributed in veins around the body via the heart. His successors suggested that veins carried blood from the head to the rest of the body, while arteries carried a subtle kind of air or spirit (shades of *chi*, perhaps).

Galen (second century AD) recognised that arteries did contain blood, but suggested that vital air or spirits travelled with it. The actual movements of the heart were not thought to be due to muscles but to the expansion of the spirits within it. In fact the heart was thought of as a mixing device to amalgamate the various spirits in the blood.

It seems extraordinary that these ideas persisted in Europe until the sixteenth century; at that time Chinese medical thinking was in many ways in advance of the European.

Again we are indebted to Dr Needham for unearthing a splendid description by a European doctor visiting China. Willen ten Rhijne (1647–1700) wrote:

> Although the Chinese physicians (who are the forerunners from whom the physicians of the Japanese borrowed the systems of healing) are ignorant in anatomy, they have nevertheless perhaps devoted more effort over many centuries to learning and teaching with very great care to the circulation of the blood, than have European physicians individually or as a group. They base the foundation of entire medicine upon the rules of the circulation, as if they were oracles of Delphi. They do not expound the rites of their art (to which they do not indiscriminately admit anyone) with honeyed words or ambiguous comparisons, nor do they obscure them with contrived and controversial nonsense, but use mechanical devices to clarify doctrinal analogy. Thus among the Chinese the masters employ hydraulic machines to demonstrate the circulation of the blood to their disciples who have earned the title of Physicians; and in the absence of such machines the masters insist on the standing of clear figures – ever paying chief honour to the authority of antiquity. The various movements of the blood must be learned through precepts and rules as laid down by the Chinese (and I promise, God willing, to present examples of these elsewhere) if a cure is to be undertaken according to their regimen.[4]

Dr Needham points out that rough measurements of the larger blood vessels had been made by the Chinese;[5] they estimated that blood had to circulate through 162 feet of blood vessels to complete one cycle. As they predicted 50 such cycles every 24 hours, during that time the total distance travelled was thought to be 8,100 feet (or 810 *chang*); this coincided with 13,500 respirations. According to their calculations blood and *chi* moved on just six inches during each individual respiration, and the time taken for one complete cycle was 28·8 minutes. (Modern studies show that the actual circulation time is only 30 seconds or so.)

Did any of these ideas reach Dr William Harvey (1578–1657) in England and prompt him to continue with his experiments? He used a hand lens to study the heart's chambers and valves in animals of many different species. His famous work *Exercitatio de motu cordis et sanguinis* was first published in 1628; it demolished the European traditional beliefs by putting forward the notion that there was a true *circulation* of blood through the organs. He suggested that blood was pumped through the system by the muscular action of the heart.

William Harvey's work was not accepted during his lifetime; for none of his contemporaries could understand how blood actually passed through the organs. In fact he was proved to be correct four years after his death. Marcello Malpighi (1628–1694) studied animal and vegetable matter under a microscope; his ambition was to be the first to study living animal tissues in the same way. In 1661 he published two letters titled *De pulmonibus* to his friend Borelli in Bologna, describing work with living frogs. Through a microscope he saw blood corpuscles passing along minute vessels (or capillaries) on the surface of the lungs and also the bladder. Malpighi showed that these were the vessels that linked arteries to veins in all the structures of the body.

Subsequent work has shown that these capillary vessels are so thin that pores appear in their lining. These allow the passage of oxygen and molecules of sugar, fat and constituents of protein and a variety of other substances required to nourish the cells. The cells exchange these nutrients for waste products which re-enter the circulation.

The microscope and cells

Malpighi continued his microscopical work and is famous for

his description of structures within the lungs, brain, kidneys and skin. Indeed, he is regarded as the father of microscopic anatomy, which revolutionised modern medicine. Doctors began to understand the importance of the cellular structure of the body: each cell, though dependent on the correct functioning of others, has its own independent role.

It was from the seventeenth century onwards that modern medicine overtook traditional Chinese studies – largely as a result of the painstaking use of the microscope. Indeed, go on a tour of a modern anatomy department today and you will find that the modern equivalent or electron microscope is usually one of the most important instruments there. In other words, doctors of the modern school realise that the more is known about the minute structures within cells, the more will be understood about the functions of tissues in health and disease. A number of important findings contributed to this idea.

Microscopical studies in the seventeenth, eighteenth and nineteenth centuries showed that all tissues, vegetable or animal, are composed of cells. Rudolf Virchow (1821–1902) was responsible for stating that all cells come from other cells (*omnis cellula e cellula*) and each type of tissue is composed of similar cells.

It became clear that generalised diseases affect some tissues more than others; for instance the growing parts of bones wherever they occur are likely to be affected by rickets when abnormal concentrations of calcium and phosphorus are present in the blood. Without a clear understanding of the underlying tissues and their functions, the treatment of rickets – to take but one example – would never have been solved in the early part of this century.

In European and Chinese medicine it was thought that the seat of disease was in the organs. Virchow's work exploded these erroneous ideas by demonstrating that it was the *cell's reaction* to abnormal conditions that was the true cause of illness.[6] Again the microscope was used in many instances to demonstrate the cell's reactions to unfavourable circumstances. Just as a captain at sea relied on his telescope, the doctors of medicine now required microscopes to scan the horizons of disease.

Diagnostic aids developed in the West

Both the Chinese and Western physicians quite rightly examined the tongue and the pulse to determine which category of disease afflicted their patients; however, in the nineteenth century a number of important additional diagnostic aids were developed in the West.[7]

Carl Wunderlich (1815–77) was perhaps the first to point out how a record of the body temperature was a guide to the precise nature and cause of infectious diseases; in 1866 the first thermometers were used in British hospitals.

The internal structure of the eye incorporating important views of blood vessels was first seen by a physician, Herman Ludwig von Helmholtz, in 1851. Four years later a Spanish singing teacher, Manuel Garcia, made the first laryngoscope for viewing the state of the larynx. Shortly after Edison's invention of electric light in 1879, the insides of many body cavities in the living patient could be seen for the first time; these included the gullet, stomach, bladder and lower bowel.

In the early 1890s various mechanical devices were designed to measure the blood pressure and record the pulse-waves in a graphic form. A major advance began in 1903 when William Einthoven of Leyden overcame enormous technical difficulties and measured the electrical changes occurring in the heart and made the first electrocardiogram.

Meanwhile the chemists were able to detect the nature and quantities of certain constituents of the blood and urine; as early as 1844, Herman von Fehling was able to measure the quantity of sugar in a diabetic patient's urine. A new branch of medicine was formed – biochemistry – which has taken an increasingly large share of a medical student's curriculum.

Yet perhaps one of the most exciting discoveries of the 1890s was the use of X-rays in medicine. Francis Williams of Boston started to examine lungs by X-rays in 1896; within a year he claimed to diagnose tuberculosis before it was detectable by any other means.[8]

Medicine had become an almost military campaign. Doctors had schooled themselves to become more soldierly in their attitude, taking decisions based on proper reconnaissance using the most appropriate and finest equipment available. No longer were they willing to accept the rules of battle against disease from revered sages of long ago. It became their habit to challenge every statement of 'fact', and refurbish old notions whenever they could. Something stated with the greatest authority but ten years before would be cast unceremoniously from medical thought, if it did not reflect the latest observations.

In this era, the idea that there were structures or channels resembling meridians running from the head to the foot (as all the foot yang meridians were meant to do) would be considered nonsense – unless there was some sensible evidence to explain it; for no one has seen such a structure in the last 400 years of dissecting cadavers. Indeed, the National Academy of Sciences in China has never found any anatomical evidence for meridians since they began their dissections in the 1920s.

Some have tried to demonstrate the existence of meridians by one means or another; for instance, in 1963, a North Korean histologist, Professor Kim Bonghan, published his discovery[9] of a system of vessels made of a tissue, never described before, which shared some similarities with both lymphatic and nerve trunks. He claimed he could demonstrate that these vessels communicated with various organs.

The Chinese Academy of Sciences was naturally interested in this discovery and sent a team of histologists to North Korea. On their return to China they were unable to repeat his experiments on Chinese cadavers. Indeed, most histologists who have seen his work regard it as spurious. Nevertheless, his work is often quoted by those who still believe in the physical existence of meridians.

Without meridians, the original model that explained acupuncture collapses completely.

A scientific view of Chinese medicine

With the scientific sails of medicine spreading so rapidly in the West, it was perhaps too easy to scoff at what appeared to be a quite unacceptable and bizarre picture of the human organism presented by the Chinese. Indeed, their intrinsically pre-Renaissance ideas of five elements are as unacceptable today as Aristotle's four.

Yet, today, many practitioners of acupuncture in the West have adopted the entire system with a few modifications and are tending to ignore the hard-won advances in medicine. To these, Khoubesserinan wrote in 1965:

> If we wish to be taken seriously, not to be confused with bone-setters and faith-healers, we must abandon the whole more or less Chinese mass of philosophy, cosmogony and mythology in which we have been entangled these 40 years past. Let us clear the decks and look at our problems without preconceived ideas. The study of anatomy and physiology of the skin, and of the central and sympathetic nervous systems, the investigation of the physico-chemical and enzymic reactions in the body, all of these should provide us with the means of solving the problem of what acupuncture really is and does.[10]

11
Scientific Trials of Acupuncture

♦

Ralph Croizier had wise words to say about the modern development of medicine in China:

> The prestige of science and the desire to build a strong, healthy nation have determined that the main thrust would be toward scientific medicine; concern with cultural continuity and vindication of a national tradition have modified the form this drive for modernization has taken. But, in the final analysis, the entire controversy over Chinese medicine has been more intellectually significant than medically important.[1]

The essential question to our minds is does acupuncture deserve an honoured place in modern medicine. Should patients brought up in a Western culture be subjected to the insertion of needles which are not attached to syringes?

Although acupuncture has been practised in Europe for at least three centuries, perhaps the most spectacular display of interest outside China has been American.

American reactions to acupuncture
The initial American reaction to acupuncture in the early 1970s was enthusiastic. When President Nixon visited China,

he took several influential physicians with him. His own physician, Dr Walter Tkach, wrote a favourable report, entitled 'I have seen acupuncture work'.[2] There was a flurry of interest amongst academic establishments. Within a year twenty-six American medical schools and universities had produced evidence for a conference, held in 1973. Their results showed that acupuncture certainly was not a panacea for all ills. Nevertheless it merited a careful study to see which diseases it might help most.

Some American experts have been distinctly cautious. Dr John Bonica, President of the International Association for the Study of Pain, made a scathing comment after a three-week visit to China in 1974: 'The claims for the high degree of efficacy of acupuncture are not based on data derived from well controlled clinical trials. In fact, in many health stations and even in some hospitals, no records are kept of either the patient's history or of his response to therapy.'[3]

The Chinese have a reply to this observation. They 'know' acupuncture works and are proud of written records going back two millennia. They could make the same comment about a Western doctor's approach to drugs such as penicillin that he 'knows' work well; most doctors do not make careful records of the effects of well-known drugs unless something untoward occurs.

Dr John Bonica decried the exploitation of Chinese medicine by unscrupulous persons who operated their 'acupuncture' centres in America, where sometimes several hundred patients were treated daily and were charged what appeared to be exorbitant fees. These centres misled the public and lured patients by their 'Madison Avenue, miracle cure' advertising. These claims were often based on short-term results in one or possibly a few patients. He concluded that he did not know of any incontrovertible scientific evidence that acupuncture was more successful than placebo therapy.[3]

What is a placebo?
Doctors using any form of treatment may cure their patients with their enthusiasm alone. According to Dr W. Houston, no drugs or remedies of any specific value were used until the mid-eighteenth century;[4] the first effective remedy was a

prescription for fresh fruit by a British Naval surgeon, James Lind, in 1753, for sailors suffering from scurvy. Until that time, in Western medicine at least, the only benefit the patient derived was from the doctor himself.

Drs Paul Lowinger and Shirlie Dobie, of the Wayne State University School of Medicine Department of Psychiatry, raised the question: 'How was it possible for a physician to hold an honored place for thousands of years in the treatment of illness if his medications were worthless? The skill of a physician was one of dealing with illness through the patient's emotions. The doctor himself was the agent by which cures occurred.'[5]

This aspect of therapy is called *placebo* (derived from the Latin – *I will please*).

The power of suggestion or placebo in relieving pain should never be underestimated. In 1955 Dr Henry Beecher, who had already written several papers about the treatment of Second World War casualties, discovered that 35 per cent of patients suffering such genuinely painful conditions as wound pain and angina derived definite relief when substances were given to them that had no pharmacological effects.[6] In other words a third of the population respond equally well to sterile saline (salt water) being injected into a vein as they would if morphine had been injected in the treatment of severe pain. In fact in the last year or so an explanation for this fascinating phenomenon has come to light and will be discussed later in the next chapter.

The powerful placebo effect has to be taken account of, when assessing new forms of treatment. Every new drug, for example, is usually submitted to trials designed to compare its effects with those of a placebo. In the assessment of a new drug patients may be split into two groups.

One group receives the placebo preparation (which looks identical to the pills containing the drug but in fact is made of chalk or some other inert substance). These patients are called the placebo group. The remainder receive the drug that is being tested. To prevent any hint of suggestion occurring between the physician and his patient, these trials are usually undertaken without either of them knowing which substance the patient is actually taking. Finally the improvement or otherwise in the patient's condition is measured by an unbiased and independent doctor, who is also unaware of which preparation is being used.

The results are carefully analysed by statistical procedures to test whether a new drug does produce 'significantly' better effects than the placebo preparation.

Clinical trials of acupuncture

In the case of acupuncture, the Chinese have found it difficult to deny patients acupuncture and offer them placebo when they think that the patient requires treatment. Indeed, they would say that this is unethical. For they already 'know' that acupuncture works. So they have not been at all keen in co-operating with the standard procedures for assessing new remedies; after all, acupuncture is hardly a new form of treatment in China. However, there are signs that they may alter this approach in the future. Nevertheless the Chinese patient knows a great deal more than his Western counterpart about acupuncture. Consequently it is more difficult to offer a Chinese patient placebo acupuncture.

It is ironic that the country that understands acupuncture best appears to be unable to participate in suitable trials for genuine ethical reasons; whilst countries where acupuncture is just beginning to be practised have a unique opportunity to assess it in a scientific manner, for many Western patients have not heard of acupuncture and are sometimes unaware that it is actually being practised upon them.

Even so, there are many difficulties in conducting trials of acupuncture in the West. In a hospital, for instance, it may be difficult to obtain patients who really do have problems; for their physicians are reluctant to advise them to have a form of treatment which they assume will not work.

Patients whose diseases are psychological

In fact many doctors who know little about the effects of acupuncture assume that it is only useful in the treatment of patients whose pains are entirely 'in the mind'. This group of patients receive as little benefit from acupuncture as they would from any other form of treatment which is not directed at the underlying emotional disorders.

**Emotionally normal patients whose X-rays, etc.,
are also normal**
On the other hand there is another group of patients who are
emotionally normal and whose X-rays and blood investigations are also normal. They are told that they have no
obvious cause for their pain – which frequently leaves them
wondering if their pains really are 'all in the mind'.

One of many examples of this group is the migraine
patient, whose head X-rays and blood investigations are
usually quite normal. A trial of the effects of acupuncture on
migraine is being carried out by British neurologists, who
prefer to remain anonymous until their work is complete.

Other members of this group of patients (those with early
arthritic pain which has not yet led to X-ray changes) are
usually excluded from trials of any kind being performed in
hospitals. Hospitals have more than enough work to cope
with patients who have marked X-ray and blood changes. Yet
this group of patients represents the majority of people suffering chronic pain. They do have causes of pain, which will be
explained later, that are not revealed by X-rays or blood tests;
they are an important group of candidates for acupuncture
therapy.

Clinical trials of acupuncture in Western hospitals
There are other formidable barriers for doctors wishing to
conduct clinical trials of acupuncture in Western hospitals.
Each well run hospital has an ethical committee, whose job is
to ensure that no research is carried out to the patients'
detriment. Usually only those patients who have already
failed to derive benefit from all the relevant Western treatment
methods are allowed to join in such a trial. For instance, a
British trial,[7] undertaken by the author and his colleagues,
showed that an almost painless form of acupuncture was
significantly more effective than placebo in relieving chronic
back pain of at least a year's duration. Some of the patients in
this trial had already undergone surgery in the back region; all
had previously failed to gain sufficient pain relief from the
conventional methods of treatment which were thought to be
appropriate.

To minimise the possibility of 'natural' recovery during treatment, patients were chosen who had been in pain for at least a year. (It is well known that many patients who have developed their illness recently recover on their own – whatever treatment is offered to them. For instance, 85 per cent of back patients recover spontaneously within eleven months.)

Finally the ethical committees often insist that these patients should continue their existing Western treatment while receiving acupuncture. After all, in their eyes the effects of acupuncture are entirely due to suggestion, until proved otherwise.

These trials, therefore, are carried out on a difficult group of patients, and inevitably the question is raised if any succeed in improving their condition: Which form of treatment is the effective one?

How should the trials be conducted?
The next problem in assessing any trial of acupuncture is the practitioner's approach to the subject.

Some practitioners of acupuncture, for instance, are convinced that the traditional legends about the subject are correct, and that modern science has not appreciated them. These practitioners may believe in the existence of the channels or meridians, already discussed in this book, and feel that they must insert their needles into the acupuncture points which are alleged to exist along the course of these structures.

In fact, this type of acupuncture is deceptively easy to study from a scientific point of view; for a computer can choose random sites on the patient's body for needling, and unbiased clinicians can readily assess the effect of using these sites as compared with placing the needles in 'acupuncture points'. Many trials of this kind have been carried out, most of which have shown little significant difference between the results obtained using 'acupuncture' points and 'placebo' or 'random' points selected by the computer.

One of the best documented trials of this type was reported by Dr Albert Gaw and his colleagues,[8] of the New England Medical Centre Hospital, Department of Psychiatry. They studied forty patients who had osteoarthritis affecting various joints.

These patients were separated into two groups. Needles were inserted into 'acupuncture' points in one group, while in the other group needles were inserted into sites nearby. Within thirty-six hours of a treatment, both groups were examined by doctors who did not know which treatment they had received. The result of this trial showed that there was no significant difference between the results obtained by inserting a needle into an 'acupuncture' point or into a 'non-acupuncture' point close by. But both groups did receive significant amounts of pain relief.

In 1973 the National Institute of Health, Bethesda, Maryland, set up a 'workshop' on the use of acupuncture in the rheumatic diseases.[9] Doctors specialising in acupuncture, medicine, neurology, psychiatry, and rheumatology met to discuss these problems. They pointed out that comparing 'true' acupuncture points with 'false' ones is not always easy, for there is no general agreement about the exact locations of acupuncture points. Many practitioners do not believe acupuncture points exist in any case. (This aspect will be described in greater detail later.) It might be important, perhaps, to standardise the size of the needle together with its depth and angle of insertion. The manner in which the needle is stimulated, either by manual twisting or by electrical apparatus, may also be an important factor.

There is no agreement between practitioners concerning the duration of individual treatments and time interval between treatments, or even the total number of treatments required. Some practitioners insist that a curious sensation called *techi* (described on page 144) should be obtained by the patient whenever a needle is inserted, while other practitioners do not feel that this is so essential. So the question which arises in every acupuncturist's mind when he reads of these trials is 'Who was the acupuncturist?', for many acupuncturists believe that they have the key to the correct practice, whereas others may not be so fortunate.

Future of acupuncture trials

As has already been described, the difficulties of running properly controlled clinical trials in an instructive manner are enormous, for the simple reason that the mechanisms of acupuncture are only just beginning to be understood and comparable placebos have not been designed.

When a little more is known about how acupuncture may work, then more informative clinical trials may be designed to test the various methods of practice.

This is an exciting stage in the development of acupuncture. The old traditional system is rapidly being dismantled by many practitioners who are racing each other to form new theories. Once a theory has been found to fit the observed phenomena, clinical trials can be conducted in a more rational framework. Such trials will be more likely to produce convincing results for or against acupuncture. Until these take place, Western sceptics will have to continue guessing whether the Chinese are practising something worthwhile or not.

Meanwhile the small band of Western doctors who are continuing to work in a field that faces the frank scepticism of their colleagues are buoyed by several thoughts.

What maintains the interest of Western doctors in acupuncture?

Dr Joseph Needham, whose scholarly approach to the history of Chinese science and medicine has already been described, believes that although scepticism is one of the important qualities in a scientist's mind it may work in two directions. He finds it hard to believe that the effects of acupuncture are entirely imaginary, when it has survived for at least two millennia and is still being practised for the benefit of at least a quarter of the world's population.

Of course fashions in medicine come and go. The practice of phlebotomy or cutting open a vein to let the blood flow was one of the Western doctors' most useful stratagems until recent times; yet today it is regarded as being worthless and in many cases dangerous. Acupuncture, on the other hand, has not only survived – despite many reverses – but is actually undergoing a renaissance today.

Those who argue that the effects of acupuncture are entirely due to placebo effects find it hard to explain how Western physicians who practise it in the treatment of chronic pain conditions can claim approximately 70 per cent success rates (whereas the maximum reported placebo success in drug trials is approximately 39 per cent).

Dr Peter Nathan, a British expert on pain – well known for his scepticism about theories that purport to explain all the mechanisms of pain – felt he had to believe what he saw when first confronted by an operation being performed under 'acupuncture anaesthesia', as it was then called, when he visited China. Although he had no explanation for the phenomenon he had just witnessed, he stated in a lecture to the Royal Society of Medicine, London, that a scientist must believe what he sees and try and find the explanation afterwards. At the end of his lecture, he was attacked by two elderly surgeons who said that 'waves of hysteria, akin to hypnosis sweep over the West every twenty-five years and this subject was the latest'. Yet, had they listened attentively, they would have heard a scientific explanation that has only just been offered in the West in the past decade.

12

Acupuncture Analgesia and the Endorphin System

We have just discussed the remarkable fact that a third of those who are in pain react as well to a placebo (pure suggestion) as to morphine. Many medical people have the illogical feeling that the good placebo reactors are more neurotic than the remaining two-thirds who were not perhaps in so much pain in the first place. Nevertheless, Dr Peter Nathan describes the placebo reactor as a doctor's 'best friend'.[1] Indeed in the past year or so, doctors have begun to understand how it is that placebo reactors are able to develop more tolerance to pain, when the right suggestions are given to them.

How does placebo work?
Drs Jon Levine, Newton Gordon and Howard Fields of the California University Department of Neurology, Physiology and Oral Surgery published an interesting account of their work with patients who reacted well to placebo in a 1978 edition of *The Lancet*.[2] They studied 51 patients who had just had their impacted wisdom teeth removed under general anaesthesia. As soon as the patients had regained consciousness they were asked to record how much pain they themselves thought they had on a special card which had a ten-centimetre line drawn upon it. A mark made at one end indicated that the patient had no pain whatsoever, while a

mark placed at the other indicated the worst possible pain that
they could imagine. Other cards were used to ask the patient if
his pain had increased, decreased or remained the same since
the last observation.

Three substances were administered in a random fashion by
injection on two occasions – two hours and three hours after
the operation – to see what effects they had on the patients'
assessments on their pain levels. The staff had no idea which
of the three substances had been given.

These three substances were placebo, morphine and
naloxone. This last substance is a drug that has the specific
property of partially blocking the effects of morphine.

The results of this trial were fascinating. As was expected,
39 per cent of patients responded well when the first injection
was placebo, while the rest remained in as much pain or more
following this injection.

The results of all those patients whose first injection was
placebo and whose second injection (given an hour later) was
naloxone were looked at carefully. The placebo reactors
stopped doing well as soon as they received naloxone; while
the pain scores of those who did not respond to placebo were
unaffected by naloxone.

This result suggested that the placebo reactors generated
some substance within their own nervous systems which not
only produced pain relief but also had the property of being
partially blocked by naloxone – that is to say, a morphine-like
substance. In other words, these patients could manufacture
their own morphine-like substance when they were given an
injection of what they thought was morphine.

This work was not just conjured out of the air. It was a
natural step based on many recent observations.

Endorphins

In the early 1970s the neurophysiological laboratories in
Shanghai reported some astonishing work performed on
rabbits. Professor Chang and his colleagues claimed that
some pain-reducing substance could be transmitted from one
animal's cerebro-spinal fluid (the solution that bathes the
brain) to another – so that when the first animal's pain
threshold was raised the second animal would respond in the

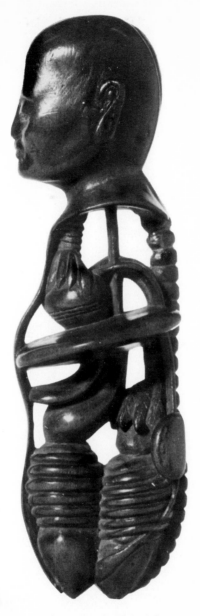

Plate 1 **Japanese box**wood model of the internal organs.

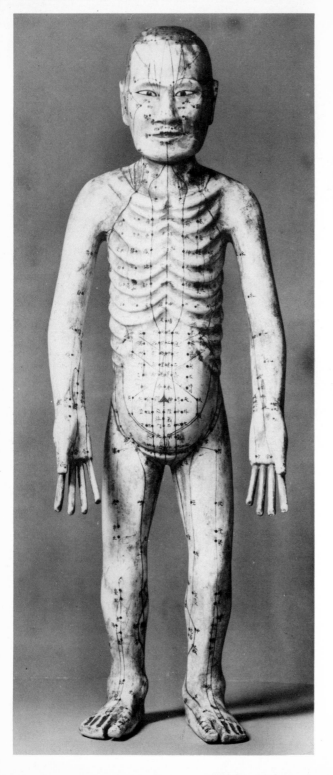

Plate 2 Papier-maché statue showing the paths of the meridians or channels.

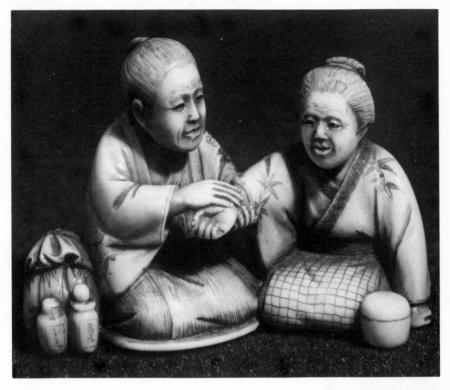

Plate 3 Japanese carved ivory figure showing the doctor's fingers on a woman's pulse; in this instance he is examining that of the ulnar artery.

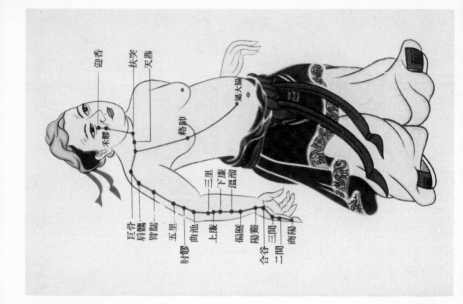

迎香
扶突
天鼎

陽大腸

絡師

禾髎

巨骨
肩髃
臂臑
肘髎
五里
曲池
上廉
三里
下廉
溫溜
偏歷
陽谿
合谷
三間
二間
商陽

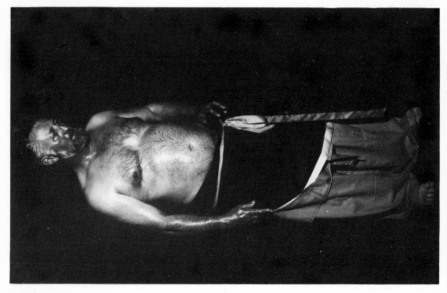

Plate 4 Highlights
travelling along the
paths of the meridians:
(a) large intestine

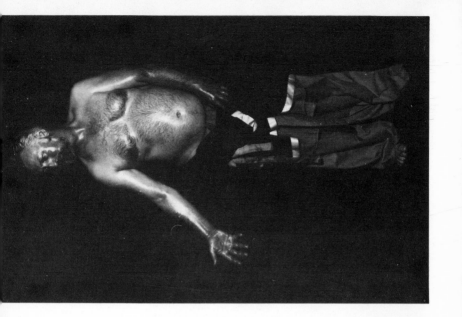

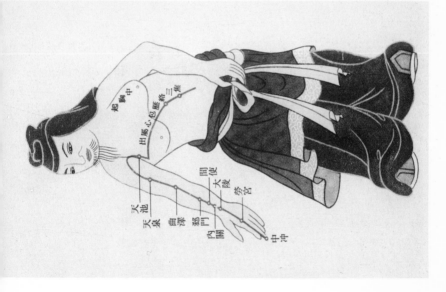

(b) pericardium.

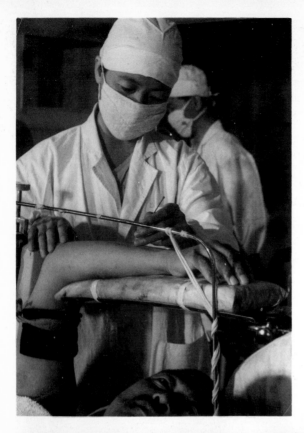

Plate 5 (a) Removal of a lung under acupuncture analgesia: twenty minutes before the operation a long needle is inserted in the patient's **forearm**.

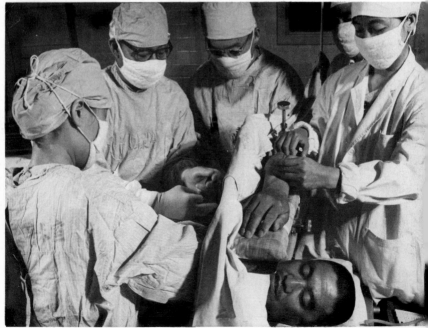

(b) **The surgeon opens up the chest – the patient still fully conscious.**

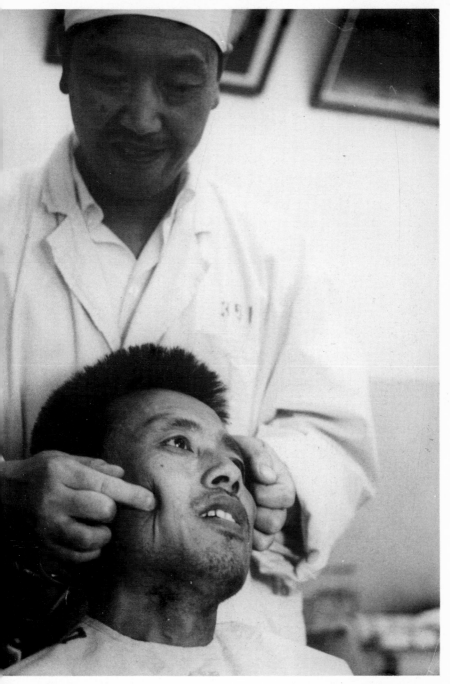

Plate 6 Acupuncture analgesia without needles – the patient's jaw muscles are being massaged so that a tooth can be extracted relatively painlessly.

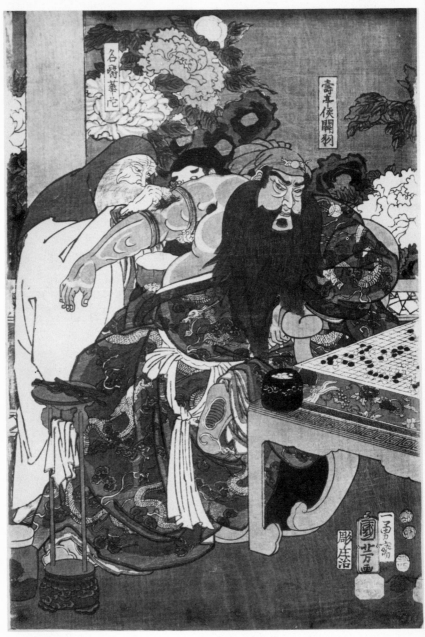

Plate 7　The famous surgeon Hua Tho operating on a war lord playing *Go.*

same fashion. It was important for these experiments that no drug should be used in the first rabbit; the Chinese answer was acupuncture.

A needle inserted into a rabbit's paw and stimulated just above its pain threshold produced an increase in the pain threshold measured on its outer ear after twenty minutes or so. As soon as this occurred, cerebro-spinal fluid was taken from this rabbit and injected into another that had not received acupuncture. The second rabbit's pain threshold also began to rise. Naloxone administered to these animals blocked these effects.

The early Shanghai experiments were greeted with disbelief by most Western and indeed many Chinese scientists until British and American studies in 1974 confirmed the fact that morphine-like substances did in fact exist in the central nervous system and many other parts of the body. These substances are called *endorphins* (the word implying *end*ogenous – produced within the body – and m*orphine*). Since these substances were isolated, an enormous amount of work has been undertaken in many pharmacological laboratories all over the world which is specifically related to the understanding of pain control. Two hundred or more chemical substances have been found in the body that behave like morphine. These are generated not only in various parts of the brain and spinal cord but also in the gut and reproductive tract. During pregnancy, for instance, the blood levels of these substances rise substantially, reaching a peak during the pain of labour. Some scientists believe that these chemicals are produced during hard times when food is scarce. Hibernating animals can be woken up by injections of naloxone, which implies that endorphins are required to alter the metabolic processes required to maintain hibernation. Similarly, congenitally fat mice lose weight when given naloxone; this suggests that over-secretion of endorphins may again slow down metabolism allowing the animal to gain too much weight.

Not producing enough endorphins is as disastrous as having too much. There is a suggestion that drug addicts who actively seek opiates produce too little of their own endorphins.

On the other hand there is a small group of people whose

production of endorphins is far too high; they do not feel pain at all. These patients cannot report the development of appendicitis at the usual early stage when most patients feel acute pain; they may rub and excoriate their eyes at night to such an extent that they may become blind through scarring, and perhaps produce large ulcers when they suck or chew their fingers in childhood. They may even sit down in open fires to warm themselves; although they are unaware of pain, they do actively seek pleasant sensations such as warmth.

The hope is that when these matters are better understood more effective therapies may become available to a whole host of patients who are either addicted, overweight or suffering pain.

However, as is usual in science, the knowledge of endorphins, scarcely a decade old, has made us realise even more than before how complicated the nervous system is; for we are now aware of entirely new systems of pain relief.

Acupuncture analgesia

One of the patients in the First Shanghai People's Hospital in 1958 suffered so much pain after his tonsils had been removed that he could not swallow. Stimulating a needle inserted into his hand in a certain location called *hegu* (see point 1, Figure 19) removed the pain so that he could eat some soft solid food called *wan tun*.[3] The doctors who were treating him wondered if post-operative pain could be treated in this way; perhaps the pain of the operation itself could be treated likewise. During the same year a tonsillectomy (surgical removal of tonsils) was performed successfully under acupuncture. The special technique required to produce sufficient pain relief for this operation was called *acupuncture anaesthesia*. However this title has been altered to *acupuncture analgesia*, as the pain relief is not total and may be likened to the partial relief achieved with morphine. Naloxone reverses this relief. This suggests that acupuncture analgesia stimulates the production of endorphins. Proof of this has been substantiated both in man and many species of animals.[4-9]

The special methods required to produce acupuncture analgesia are interesting. The needles are usually inserted deeply into muscle, preferably over their motor points (an area which is most likely to produce muscle contractions when stimulated electrically). Strong manual or electrical stimulation is required to produce painful sensations. These must be continued for at least fifteen or twenty minutes for the analgesia to occur; any shorter period of time does not have this effect. If the stimulation is continued for ninety minutes or more, the effects are reversed; in other words the patient develops a 'tolerance' to the acupuncture analgesia.[10]

Where the needles are inserted

When acupuncture analgesia was first investigated by the Chinese, they thought that as many needles as possible should be tried for each operation; sometimes a hundred needles were used for resection of a lung. Many of the needles were inserted in corresponding 'channels or meridians' according to the traditional theories.

Experiments were started on the medical staff and other healthy volunteers; gradually they excluded ineffective sites. Over the course of a few years they established approximately forty-four most commonly used points (see Figure 19).[11] Each operation required a combination of points selected from these forty-four. On the whole as few needles as possible are used at any one time; for they found that few needles were more effective than many. Sometimes the same combination of points is used for two different operations; usually the two operations in this case are in the same region of the body. Thus a combination required for tonsillectomy might be the same as one required for tooth extraction.

Response to acupuncture analgesia

There are regions of the body that respond poorly to acupuncture analgesia; they lie on the limbs – below the elbows and knees. On the other hand there are parts of the body that have a higher success; the upper parts of the body and particularly the neck are relatively responsive – thus tooth extractions and removal of the thyroid glands are frequently carried out under acupuncture analgesia. In the case of tooth extractions some centres in China use no needles at all (see Plate 6); the patient receives deep massage to the muscles around the jaw during the procedure. The advantage of performing neck operations

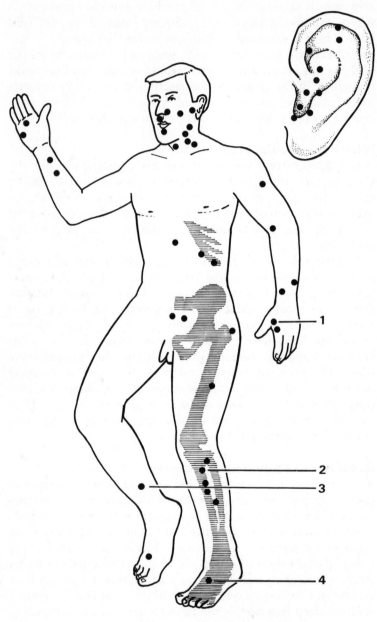

Figure 19   *The points most commonly used for acupuncture analgesia.*

without general anaesthesia is that the patient can talk during the operation – thus demonstrating that the very delicate nerves to his larynx have not been damaged.

The other advantages of performing operations under acupuncture analgesia have been summarised by Drs Lu Gwei-Djen and Joseph Needham:[12]

1   No deaths have ever been reported from acupuncture analgesia; intrinsically it is a very safe procedure compared with the use of drugs and gases required to produce general anaesthesia.

2   There is no interference with the regulatory systems of the body; while general anaesthesia often interferes, for example, with the control of respiration and blood pressure, and the functions of the brain, bowels and kidneys.

3   There are less of the post-operative complications, which sometimes occur after general anaesthesia – nausea, urinary retention (where the patient is unable to pass urine), constipation and infections of the respiratory tract.

Drs Lu Gwei-Djen and Joseph Needham described their first experience of seeing such operations: 'In July 1972 we found ourselves in the surgical department of the Second General Hospital of Chungsham Medical College at Canton, about to join the growing and by now very large number of Western surgeons, physicians and men of science, who have personally witnessed major operations under acupuncture analgesia.'[13] They described how a country girl aged twenty-four had a Caesarian section performed under acupuncture analgesia; it was her first pregnancy and the baby was not lying in the correct position – furthermore she had a double uterus and her pelvis was too small. She lay on her back and remained calm and impassive throughout the procedure, and showed no signs of pain even during the extraction of the child. The analgesia that she obtained had no deleterious effect on the baby. The only pain relief she received was from the manipulation of two needles inserted into each leg, one a little below the knee (see point 2, Figure 19) and the other (point 3) a hand's-breadth above the inner aspect of the ankle.

Towards the end of the operation two further needles were inserted into her ears to augment the effects of those placed in her legs.

The same authors also witnessed an inch-long stone being removed from a 57-year-old sailor's upper ureter (the vessel that conducts urine from the kidney). Here only four needles were used: one in his back just above the incision in his loin; another was inserted in his front just below the wound; yet another was inserted into *hegu* on the hand (see point 1, Figure 19); while the last needle was inserted into the foot between the first and second toes (see point 4). During the procedure some of the needles were stimulated electrically, producing muscle contractions, while the others were continuously moved about by the anaesthetist to make sure that the nerve receptors were adequately stimulated. The patient displayed no sign of pain or deep malaise, and did not wince at the incision or at any other time.

They also met a patient who had part of his lung removed under acupuncture analgesia (an example of this is shown in Plate 5); he had felt no pain and was enjoying a good appetite immediately afterwards. Later they witnessed three other procedures: a harelip repair operation, a removal of a con-genital cyst from a thyroid, and – perhaps the most impressive operation of all – a large bone tumour being removed with a thread-saw from a forty-year-old man's jaw.

Disadvantages of acupuncture analgesia
At this stage the disadvantages of acupuncture analgesia should be thought about. Certain painful experiences are not blocked as well as others – particularly extremes of heat and cold, and tissues being squeezed or stretched. Handling of internal organs must be kept to a minimum to avoid nausea and shock. When operations are being performed in the abdomen while using general anaesthesia, curare is given to paralyse the muscles; no such relaxation occurs with acupunc-ture analgesia. Thus, much of the success of an operation depends on the skills of the surgeon. In China the surgeons have to be quick and deft; in fact they are known as the 'flying knives'.

In order to initiate acupuncture analgesia the patient has to be subjected to painful needling for at least twenty minutes. Those who can tolerate this without becoming anxious are much more likely to undergo an operation successfully, using this form of pain relief. Children, for example, are not usually suitable as few will tolerate such severe needling, and keep still during major surgery. Indeed, animals undergoing operations under acupuncture analgesia have to be tied down firmly (see Figure 20, page 126).

Most operations carried out under acupuncture analgesia have to be performed in less than an hour; as has been said before the patient may develop tolerance to the needling after 90 minutes or so.

How many patients can benefit from acupuncture analgesia?

The most obvious question that springs to a Western doctor's mind is, What is the actual success rate? Table 7 gives the results of the pain relief obtained in 80,000 operations[14] performed under acupuncture analgesia in various hospitals in China.

Table 7   *Reactions of patients during operation under acupuncture analgesia*

Group	Reaction	%
Group I (excellent)	Calm. Slightest sensation of pain only. (Monitoring of pulse, respiration and blood pressure revealed no significant changes.)	37·3
Group II (good)	Occasional groaning. Dull pain experienced. (Slight changes revealed in physiological data.)	38·5
	Total	75·8
Group III (fair)	Definitely in pain, but not demanding general anaesthesia. (More marked changes in monitored data.)	15·4
Group IV (poor)	Requires general anaesthesia. (Very marked deterioration in physiological data.)	8·8

Here we can see the percentage success of various categories of patients. All patients had their blood pressures and the rates of their respiration and pulse monitored during the operation, for pain usually affects all three. The patient's requests were also taken into account.

According to these figures the two most successful groups, I and II, totalled 75·8 per cent; in other words at least three-quarters (or 60,640) of these patients did well.

However, what is just as interesting is the remarkably high figure in group III, representing 15·4 per cent or just over a sixth (12,320) of the patients who were definitely in pain yet not demanding general anaesthesia. How many patients in the West would undergo major surgery in a painful manner without demanding general anaesthesia? There must have been some special factors at work with this group of Chinese patients: perhaps they were trying very hard to make the experiment work and not let their doctors down, or were actually more frightened of a general anaesthetic; in some instances they may have developed the pain at an advanced stage in the operation, when it would have been technically difficult to induce general anaesthesia; or the general anaesthetic facilities may just not have been available at all in some centres at that time.

We are all well aware that almost any assertion in medicine can be 'proved' by statistics: George Bernard Shaw quipped that the wearing of a gold watch could be shown to be a good protection against tuberculosis.

The first question the Western investigator should ask about Table 7 is whether these figures represent the total population of patients who had surgery during a particular period of time or whether they were drawn from a specially selected group of patients. In other words, in this table, were all surgical patients given acupuncture analgesia first and did only those in group IV (8·8 per cent or 7,040) receive a general anaesthetic?

As far as we in the West could tell, that table could not represent the total population of patients who had surgery, as our own efforts to repeat the procedures produced very different results. Dr Felix Mann published a paper in a 1974 edition of the *British Journal of Anaesthesia*.[15] Here he conducted a hundred trials of acupuncture analgesia in thirty-five subjects, and found that only 10 per cent of cases developed adequate analgesia for a surgical operation to be performed; in

65 per cent mild analgesia occurred which was insufficient for surgery; and in the remaining 25 per cent there was only minimal analgesia.

He commented that the degree of stimulus used was so intense that the resulting pain would be unacceptable to most Western patients.

This article made Dr Mann unpopular with many Western practitioners who were unwilling to look at acupuncture critically in a scientific manner. Yet recent unpublished figures from China agree with Dr Mann's and accept the fact that acupuncture analgesia is of benefit to 10–15 per cent only of the total population of patients requiring surgery.

Selection of patients

What apparently happens is that patients are screened on arrival in hospital a few days before the operation. First of all, only patients who volunteer for acupuncture analgesia are accepted. These are then given a 'trial' of acupuncture analgesia. It is now known that those who tolerate the severe needling required with equanimity will make the best subjects; while those who flinch or become agitated may safely be excluded from having it performed on the operating table, especially in front of a team of sceptical Western doctors.

The actual effects of the acupuncture analgesia are gauged as far as possible in advance. Stimuli that would normally hurt the patient are applied to the site of the operation after twenty minutes or so's strong needling in the ward, and if the patient no longer reacts in the usual way then it might be safe to assume that this form of pain relief may be an adequate provision for the operation itself.

Finally the patient has to have the operation explained to him at some length, as he will be conscious throughout it and will be able to feel what is going on without, he hopes, the associated pain. The patient's co-operation with the surgeon is therefore imperative.

Many patients receive sedative and pain-relieving drugs before the operation. Local anaesthetics are frequently employed to allow the surgeon to cut through the skin and other painful regions, or to block cough reflexes in lung operations. Many surgeons throughout the world perform similar operations on conscious patients with the same agents without having recourse to acupuncture analgesia at all; but the Chinese would reply that acupuncture analgesia reduces the amount of such drugs required in appropriate patients.

The exact number of surgical patients who are not offered acupuncture analgesia for their operations is not known; but, if Table 7 is correct and 10–15 per cent of the total population of surgical patients derive benefit from acupuncture analgesia, then 81–87 per cent of patients are excluded from the trial for one reason or another.

As in all medical matters, initial enthusiasm for a new discovery can carry events too far. It was perhaps tempting to use this sensational form of pain relief to attract world-wide attention to China and to the special knowledge that she had in this field, particularly during a period of political turmoil where scientists were not considered to be important – during the Cultural Revolution (1966–76).

It is interesting to note that the Chinese have publicly confessed that Western visitors were deliberately hoodwinked during the 1960s and early 1970s. A 1980 edition of the British newspaper the *Daily Telegraph*[16] reported an article from the Shanghai newspaper *Wen Hui Bao* of similar date: this revealed that acupuncture analgesia had become a political instrument of the Cultural Revolution. The report went on to say that many doctors and patients during those years of radical rule were forced to use the acupuncture method, regardless of its effectiveness, because of the 'political needs of the time'; even when the patients wanted to scream, they were only allowed to shout political slogans; doctors who objected to the use of acupuncture analgesia on unsuitable patients were denounced as counter-revolutionaries and handed over to the masses for criticism.

Certainly the false impressions created by figures published at that time may have a long-lasting deleterious effect on the Western scientific community; yet those who have visited or spoken to Chinese scientists in recent times have been impressed by their careful and sincere observations.

Is acupuncture analgesia a form of hypnosis?
In the same issue of the *Daily Telegraph*, the paper's medical

correspondent suggested there may well be an element of hypnosis, suggestibility or faith operating in those who respond well to acupuncture analgesia. This idea has obviously occupied the minds of scientists, as there are numerous records of operations being performed under hypnosis alone.

Dr Basil Finer, a British anaesthetist, working in Uppsala, Sweden, has written a fascinating report, 'Mental Mechanisms in the Control of Pain',[17] that outlines present thinking on this subject. Here he describes Indian work in the mid-nineteenth century; in one hospital almost all the surgery was conducted under hypnotic analgesia.[18] Hospital auxiliaries sat in front of their patients sometimes for six hours at a stretch, blowing lightly on their foreheads and making hypnotic passes – a method quite different from that employed in acupuncture analgesia. What interested Dr Finer was that the number of reported cases of gangrene from operations conducted in this way was very low (a mere 5 per cent); while at the same time in the West (before Lister introduced antisepsis with carbolic acid) half the patients who underwent surgery died of gangrene afterwards.

Those who support acupuncture analgesia also claim less infection following its use.[19] However, here the similarities between acupuncture and hypnotic analgesia cease.

Differences between acupuncture and hypnotic analgesia

One of the main differences between acupuncture and hypnotic analgesia is the behaviour of the subject. In man, the subject is in an altered state of consciousness when hypnotised. James Esdaile, the East India Company Surgeon, who performed the operations under hypnosis that have just been described, noted that the patients were in a sleep-like trance and were not able to co-operate with him; but patients are quite able to co-operate and talk sensibly to the surgeon when given acupuncture analgesia.

In animals hypnosis engenders complete passivity and immobility; this is often called a 'death feint'. The animal undergoing acupuncture analgesia is absolutely alert and quite able to spring nimbly off the operating table or bite the surgeon; in fact it has to be tied down to prevent this happening (see Figure 20).

Three reports suggest that the endorphin system is not employed in hypnotic analgesia, for the drug naloxone does not apparently affect hypnotic states.[20–22] (However, it is fair to say that there is one account which says the opposite.[23])

Perhaps the most telling evidence that the effects of acupuncture on raising pain thresholds are not due to suggestion or hypnosis was shown by Dr Chang Chen-Yü and his colleagues in 1973.[24] Here the pain thresholds were determined in volunteers. The thresholds were determined

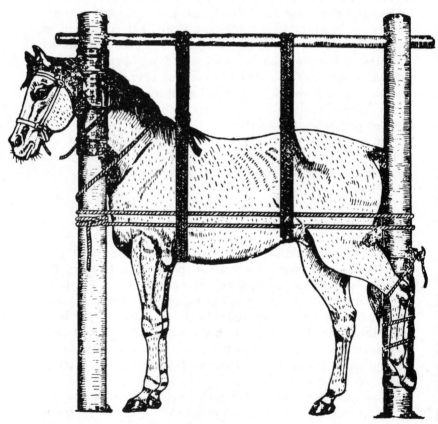

Figure 20   *A horse being tethered firmly before acupuncture analgesia is performed.*

again after a quarter of an hour of (a) rest, (b) acupuncture applied to needles inserted deep into muscles, (c) similar acupuncture following local anaesthetic blockade of the nerves supplying the skin, and finally (d) acupuncture following local anaesthetic blockade of the muscle as well. The pain threshold was raised by procedures (b) and (c) only; but once the nerve receptors had been blocked both in the skin and muscle, as occurred in (d), then the pain thresholds remained unaltered. This strongly suggests that acupuncture's effects are mediated initially through the direct effect of the needles on the peripheral nervous system, whereas the effects of hypnosis probably start in the higher centres of the brain.

If we accept that acupuncture analgesia employs certain pathways through the central nervous system that involve the endorphin system, while the hypnotic analgesia operates through other as yet unknown systems, then it seems possible that the combination of the two would increase the likelihood of success. It is interesting to conjecture that acupuncture analgesia conducted on animals may in fact be achieving this unwittingly; for placing an animal under restraint can itself induce hypnosis. Thus, binding the animal down before carrying out surgery under acupuncture analgesia may augment its success by hypnosis. Similarly in man, during the Cultural Revolution, giving the patient Chairman Mao's thoughts to read during the operation may have had similar effects.

The future of acupuncture analgesia
At present, the low success rate and difficulties in predicting which patient will perform well with acupuncture analgesia makes it an unacceptable form of pain relief for major surgery in the West. However, the fact that 10–15 per cent of patients do derive substantial relief from acupuncture analgesia is in itself a phenomenon worthy of investigation, for such studies might unveil new methods of pain relief which may prove extremely useful, particularly when drugs may prove dangerous as can sometimes occur in obstetrics.

13
Conditions that Have Been Treated by Acupuncture Therapy

◆

In the previous chapter we considered acupuncture *analgesia* for the relief of pain during major surgery. However, the majority of practitioners in the West are interested only in relieving chronic conditions; the form of acupuncture they use is called acupuncture *therapy*. They employ a more gentle and less painful technique in order to contribute to a patient's long-term recovery from an illness (often in combination with other forms of appropriate treatment).

The question we would like to discuss is which illnesses can be relieved by acupuncture therapy. There have been enormous problems in answering this question satisfactorily.

Dr Bernard Millman, of the Department of Anesthesia at Stanford University Medical School, California, wrote a very thoughtful review of this subject in 1977.[1] He described veterinary work showing how arthritis and back problems in horses and dogs could be managed by acupuncture therapy. This seemed to show that acupuncture was not entirely humbug; however, the susceptibility of human beings to psychological manipulation was extremely difficult to eliminate from scientific trials of so idiosyncratic and physical a form of treatment.

Dr Millman's message appeared to be that the method itself is not so important as the psychological effect that it engenders. He stressed how trials of new methods of treatment that have not been exposed to scientific assessment often appear to have an 80–90 per cent success rate in the mind of an over enthusiastic practitioner; while under scientifically controlled conditions these results would be reduced to 30 per cent or so if they were entirely due to suggestion. At that time his view was that the results of acupuncture followed this trend. (However, as we will see in Chapter 14, a properly conducted clinical trial of acupuncture therapy performed in the West suggests that it has a significantly higher success than 30 per cent.)

Dr Millman reminded the reader that the most likely patients to respond to suggestion are those suffering anxiety; many apparent remissions from illness can be directly caused by relieving mental stress, rather than by any particular system of treatment.

Beneficial psychological effects
Certainly many patients feel rested and relaxed after receiving acupuncture therapy; a few even drift off to sleep during a treatment. Some may feel as though their whole body, and particularly those parts that were in pain, is glowing with warmth and ease. Following a successful course of treatment, patients may feel a new lease of 'energy' and immediately undertake work they were too ill to contemplate before.

On rare occasions the patient's entire character may appear to change. I remember a large, full-bearded ship's captain who was known for his somewhat ticklish temper; he was treated for an old-standing pain in the side of his chest. After two treatments (which merely consisted of inserting two small needles into a region of his back for a few seconds) his wife and crew noticed the most amazing change in his behaviour: he lost all his pain and became quite jovial; in fact, he appeared to mellow overnight.

Unhappily, the majority of patients do not improve so briskly; their way forward is all too slow and lacking in drama. Nevertheless, their progress, as one might expect, is usually mirrored by reduced anxiety and tension.

If Dr Bernard Millman is correct in his inference that acupuncture's benefits are entirely attributable to such psychological improvement, then we might ask how acupuncture therapy causes them. It is probably a 'chicken-and-egg' story.

When a long-standing pain is relieved by any form of treatment, a patient would expect to feel considerably less 'tense'. If, on the other hand, a treatment succeeds in making a patient feel more relaxed, then he would expect to be in less pain as well. Here the traditional Chinese physicians have made a valuable contribution to medicine; for they rarely appear to make a distinction between the 'body' and 'mind'. Most things that affect the body affect the mind also, and vice versa.

Perhaps the acupuncturist's attitude and approach are better altogether at providing relief from stress during treatment than those of his Western-trained counterpart. Yet the Western approach is necessary also.

Professor Kumio Yamachita, of the Department of Anaesthesia, National Medical Centre Hospitals of Tokyo, summed this idea up rather well:

> I believe that Western medicine may be likened to a father's love, strict and at times severe; and Oriental medicine to a mother's love, gentle and patient. Neither one parent's love, nor one school of medicine is complete in itself; they need to be combined, to become a larger whole. The combination, Western-Oriental medicine, like God's love, is the ideal *par excellence*.[2]

Conditions suggested by lay practitioners of acupuncture

In many countries outside the People's Republic of China, non-medically trained practitioners use acupuncture extensively and describe a variety of treatable conditions that far exceeds any list drawn up by more cautious Western-trained doctors.

Many practitioners of acupuncture who have not received a full medical training rely totally on the traditional Chinese ideas that disease is apparently caused by an 'imbalance' or disordered flow of the imaginary substance *chi* – described in Chapter 2 as a symbolic form of 'life-force' or 'vital energy'. Some of these practitioners may believe, quite sincerely, that they alone understand how to adjust and 'rebalance' the flow of *chi*, and tell the patient that the healing effects of a perfect circulation of *chi* have to be restored before the illness is resolved. They may warn the patient that this 'process' some-times requires regular treatments given over a space of several months or even years before a satisfactory improvement in his condition is noticed.

Even people who are not ill at all in the conventional sense of the word may receive treatment from a practitioner of traditional Chinese medicine; for the work of a 'superior' physician was thought to be principally in the treatment of disease in its earliest phase, before it became gross enough to declare itself to the patient.[3] The effectiveness of this Utopian and very worthy idea has, unfortunately, not been proven.

In other words, practically any disease either in the present or the future is potentially 'treatable' by acupuncture, pro-vided both the practitioner and the patient accept the tenets of traditional Chinese medicine – as interpreted by a non-Chinese non-Western-trained person. Such a list appears to include cancer and even some venereal diseases.[4,5]

Exaggerated claims

In Great Britain, an island bastion of conservative medicine, exaggerated claims have done little for acupuncture's de-velopment. An editorial in a 1973 edition of the *British Medical Journal* described the history of acupuncture in Britain from the early nineteenth century. It ended with a statement:

> Acupuncture is said to have been devised . . . to re-establish in the patient a correct equilibrium between the *Yang*, or the male element, and the *Yin*, or female element. While this worthy motive appears never to have been challenged, the variety of explanations for its *modus operandi*, the com-plexity of the techniques, its exploitation by charlatans . . . and above all its built-in association with the occult seems weighed heavily against its chances of thorough trial by medical scientists faced with competing claims of seem-ingly greater priority.[6]

Treatable conditions suggested by doctors in the West
Most practitioners who have had a full medical training are
able to take a more reasoned and cautious approach to the
subject, as they are so aware of the efficacy of many conventional Western remedies. Therefore Western-trained doctors would only consider acupuncture as a justifiable form of
treatment for those conditions which do not often gain long-
term relief from more conventional remedies. The relief of
chronic pain is an excellent example and is described in more
detail in Chapter 17.

Conditions treated in China
However, in China acupuncture has been used for an
enormous variety of conditions.

An excellent account of the number of conditions considered treatable by acupuncture is to be found in a handbook
written by the Shanghai City Acupuncture and Moxibustion
Research Laboratory in 1971. This work is translated into
English by Dr Hans Ågren, of the University Department of
Uppsala, Sweden.[7] It contains descriptions of the acupuncture
treatment of a Pandora's box of maladies from schizophrenia
to gangrene. Infectious diseases, such as malaria, were also included.

Other more recent Chinese sources describe the treatment
of angina (pain associated with the heart), coronary heart
disease and also abnormal rhythms of the heart.[8]

It is important to point out at this stage that *before* a patient
seeks acupuncture for any serious condition he should consult
his own doctors or specialists first; only then can the treatment
be properly assessed. It would be quite wrong to imagine that
an acupuncturist who is *not* also a cardiologist (heart specialist)
could possibly decide on his own whether or not acupuncture
was an appropriate form of treatment for a particular patient's
coronary heart disease, for example.

Another example of problems which should be referred to
Western-trained specialists are those associated with pregnancy; these include morning sickness, prolonged labour,
correcting the position of the baby within the womb (including a breech presentation), and failure to produce enough milk

following delivery. The treatment of all of these with acupuncture has been discussed in China.[9]

Can addiction be treated?

To this growing list of conditions, acupuncture has been used for the relief of addiction to a variety of substances including tobacco, hashish, heroin, cocaine, alcohol and barbiturates. This work began in Hong Kong in the early 1970s when Dr H. L. Wen, a neurosurgeon, noted that drug addicts tended to lose their withdrawal symptoms while receiving acupuncture; apparently the most effective method was to stimulate electrically a needle inserted into the outer ear. Many centres in the world have been financed to continue this work. In Britain Margaret Patterson, a missionary surgeon, who has worked with Dr Wen, is pioneering many developments in this field; her book *Addictions can be cured* describes her early ideas about this new method of treatment, which she now calls neuro-electric therapy (NET).[10]

Using acupuncture to relieve an addict's withdrawal symptoms may be part of the endorphin story, described in Chapter 13; it is suggested that we are producing endorphins or morphine-like substances within our own brains and perhaps the addict has a faulty production of these substances and craves injections of morphine or heroin and so forth to replace them. Another theory suggests that the addict may damage his own secretion of endorphins by excessive use of drugs and that when these drugs are suddenly denied him he has too little endorphin production of his own – hence the agony of his withdrawal symptoms.

We also know that endorphin production can be increased by acupuncture stimulation; a 1979 study carried out jointly in Hong Kong and St Bartholomew's Hospital, London, showed that concentrations of some but not all of the endorphins were raised by acupuncture in heroin addicts during the withdrawal period and furthermore their symptoms were successfully suppressed at the same time.[11] (The same team – Drs Vicky Clement-Jones, Lorraine McLoughlin, Susan Tomlin, G. M. Besser, Lesley Rees and H. L. Wen – demonstrated in the following year that the levels of other endorphins were raised following acupuncture

therapy given for the relief of chronic pain;[12] they suggested
that this form of treatment may operate through many pathways in the nervous system at the same time.)

Guiding the addict through the withdrawal stage from his
drugs is only a small fraction of the treatment. The most
difficult part is to change his attitude so that he does not seek
drugs again; this requires knowledge and skills in the practitioner far beyond the art of acupuncture. In other words, a
patient who seeks acupuncture from a practitioner unversed
in the intricacies of the addict's world will not receive the
support he needs once his withdrawal symptoms have been
resolved. If this new form of treatment becomes a popular
method amongst doctors it should be practised in special
centres or surroundings where the patient receives all the
other forms of special attention he needs.

Treatable conditions suggested by WHO delegates

In 1979, the World Health Organisation (WHO) held a meeting in Peking to discuss acupuncture; doctors practising
acupuncture therapy in many different countries were asked
to discuss the most likely conditions that might benefit from
its use.

Dr Bannerman, the WHO programme manager for traditional medicine, reported a bewildering variety of illnesses
that the delegates felt could be treated in this way.[13]

The delegates were asked to include illnesses that they had
treated successfully by acupuncture therapy. This list was not
necessarily derived from formal clinical trials conducted in a
scientific manner; the difficulties of carrying out such trials
have already been discussed. They were also anxious to include a note that because a particular disease was mentioned it
did not indicate the efficacy of acupuncture therapy in its
relief.

The WHO delegates' list included upper respiratory tract
infections such as sinusitis, acute tonsillitis, and chronic nasal
conditions. They went on to describe the treatment of acute
bronchitis and bronchial asthma (a disease characterised by
wheezing when the spasm of tubes or bronchae within the
lung prevents the patient from breathing out properly). They
believed that treatment for asthma was most effective in

children and in patients without any other complications in the lung.

They felt that gastro-intestinal disorders, such as peptic ulcers and colitis, could be treated. They even described the treatment of facial paralysis or palsy, particularly in the first three to six months of the condition (see p. 156 for a critical comment on this matter). Some improvements in movements of motor function in patients who have had strokes or who have had poliomyelitis were also reported; these findings should also be questioned.

They discussed a variety of painful conditions such as tennis elbow, frozen shoulder, chronic back pain and sciatica and osteoarthritis as being suitable for acupuncture therapy. These conditions will be discussed in more detail in Chapters 14 and 17.

To what extent and in what possible manner acupuncture therapy can be expected to contribute to the relief of these diseases will be discussed in succeeding chapters. After all, a needle on its own has no effect; it is the patient's reaction to its insertion that is important.

The vital question
Doctors, trained in the West, who have just begun to employ acupuncture therapy and are using their conventional medical approach to their patients as much as ever before, often find therapeutic results (be they psychological or 'physical') that they would never have obtained if a needle had not been inserted; in other words, apart from that one act alone, their methods of investigating, examining and advising the patient have remained unaltered.

What has the insertion of a mere needle done to achieve an effect that is often not obtainable in the same patient even when he has already been offered long periods of drug regimens and other more conventional Western remedies at the behest of the same doctor or perhaps when his colleagues employ a similar amount of care and concern?

14
The Needle Effect

◆

Western doctors have called the patient's reaction to the insertion of the needle on its own the 'needle effect'. Indeed, Professor Karel Lewit (Department of Vertebrogenic Disorders, the Central Railway Health Institute, Prague, Czechoslovakia) decided to investigate the effects of inserting a needle.[1]

He used the smallest and finest needles that were long enough to reach the structures required. In the neck region where all tissues lie close to the skin he was able to use acupuncture needles. In the lower back he used thin lumbar puncture needles to reach deeper regions. As no drugs or other substances were injected into these patients, this technique was described as 'dry' needling.

Between 1975 and 1976, he reviewed 241 patients suffering chronic pain coming from their muscles, tendons or ligaments. Some of these patients had pains in more than one region of their bodies. In all, 312 pain sites were studied. The pain in 270 (or 86·8 per cent) of these 312 sites was relieved immediately by 'dry' needling.

Professor Karel Lewit managed to review 245 of the sites where pain was successfully relieved: 32 patients (13·1 per cent of the successful group) had relief of pain for several days only; while 213 patients (86·9 per cent of this group) had pain relief lasting several weeks or more; in fact no less than 92 (or 37·5 per cent) had permanent relief of tenderness apparently from one treatment.

A description of one of his patients who derived partial relief in this way indicates that at least some had severe disorders:

A 46-year-old male technician had a scar in his back caused by suppuration (or collection of pus) in childhood. At the time of examination he could not walk without the aid of sticks and had a number of deformities and curvatures in his back and pelvic region. In addition, a special X-ray examination revealed a massive protrusion of one of his discs in the lower back.

The most tender region was around the scar that he had had since childhood. 'Dry' needling of this region was intensely painful; but immediately afterwards the curvature in his spine disappeared and he could walk without sticks. However, to give him complete relief of pain at a later date, local anaesthetic had to be injected into his spinal region. Therefore in this instance 'dry' needling was augmented by more conventional procedures; nevertheless, the reported fact remains that this patient was able to walk unaided immediately following the insertion of one needle into his back, despite the manifest disabilities he had beforehand.

Professor Karel Lewit stressed that 'dry' *needling* should often be combined with other forms of therapy, otherwise relapses would occur unless all other causes of the pain had been removed.

Ah Shi points

The idea of needling tender spots is not new: in the Tang dynasty (AD 618–907) a famous Chinese physician, Sun Szu-miao, advanced a similar thesis;[2] his maxim was, 'Puncture wherever there is tenderness.' The Chinese call such tender regions *Ah Shi* points; *Ah Shi* means 'Oh Yes'. A patient says this politely when he feels the severe pain caused by the physician finding the right spot and pressing on it with his finger. In other words, both the patient and the doctor have to co-operate to find these regions.

The effects of random needling

Most human beings (and we include doctors amongst their number) enjoy working to a routine with certain rules and regulations; they would feel unhappy if they thought none were required in their work. Those practising acupuncture are not exceptional in this. Traditionally trained practitioners abide by a complex code that has been elaborated over many centuries, and are not free to experiment boldly. Western-trained doctors who use acupuncture have greater liberty in this subject; but even they often feel obliged to use a hotch-potch of traditional and modern ideas – without really deciding which are the effective requirements for the success of the treatment.

Therefore a trial carried out by Drs Charles Godfrey and Peter Morgan in the Department of Rehabilitation, The Wellesley Hospital, Toronto, and the Department of Preventive Medicine and Biostatics of the University of Toronto, came like a bolt from the blue.[3]

They studied patients who all complained of chronic dull, constant, moderately severe pain in various parts of their bodies; their diagnoses included a number of common complaints associated with pain – such as tennis elbow, neck or back strain, degenerated spinal or intervertebral discs, and various osteoarthritic conditions. (Any patients with active disease processes attacking their joints or who were suspected of having other more serious conditions that might be responsible for their pain were excluded from the trial.)

These conditions were satisfied by 193 patients and they were included in the trial. The purpose of the study was to observe the difference in results, if any, between those associated with 'properly' carried out acupuncture and those obtained when the same needles were inserted in a similar manner into an 'inappropriate' part of the body; for instance, if a patient had a shoulder problem, the 'proper' acupuncture would be carried out in the shoulder region – while the 'inappropriate' acupuncture would be performed as far away as possible near the opposite ankle.

The 'proper' acupuncture was performed by a suitably qualified Chinese doctor, trained in the Shanghai Second Medical College; he had left the People's Republic of China, was a lecturer in the Department of Physiology at Hong Kong University and happened to be on sabbatical leave in Toronto.

The 'inappropriate' acupuncture was carried out by other

members of the department. The patient lay on his back, and a screen was arranged so that he could not see who was carrying out either form of acupuncture.

The only communication between the practitioner and the patient was via a third person. When 'inappropriate' acupuncture was being performed, this third party would explain that the reason why it was being carried out so far away from the site of the pain was that it produced its effects via linking 'channels' or 'meridians'.

Another member of the team was a doctor who did not know which treatment the patient had received; his duty was to assess the patient's condition both before the course of treatment began and at various times during and after the treatment. The results of the trial were based entirely on the observations of this impartial medical witness.

The final results were not expected – at least by those who favour the idea that acupuncture does not have any effect other than by suggestion, or by those who think that the rules and regulations of acupuncture adopted by the Chinese doctor involved in the trial were absolutely necessary for its practice:

1 There was no significant difference between the results obtained by the two groups; that is, whether acupuncture was applied in a 'proper' or 'inappropriate' manner made no difference to the results.
2 60 per cent of both groups were successfully relieved of their pain.

If the results of acupuncture were entirely attributable to suggestion, as Dr Bernard Millman suggested in Chapter 6, the results of both groups should have been approximately 30 per cent; thus the 60 per cent figure shown in this trial indicated that acupuncture offers something more than suggestion.

The fact that 'inappropriate' acupuncture was as successful as the 'proper' acupuncture suggested that random needling may be successful in relieving pain.

Another valuable investigation, this time carried out in rats, confirmed both of these possibilities in more detail.

The diffuse noxious inhibitory control system

In the INSERM laboratories in Paris, Drs Daniel Le Bars, Anthony Dickenson and Jean-Marie Besson made a discovery in 1979[4] which may prove to be another vital step to the understanding of acupuncture and many other methods of relieving pain. They wanted to know if a painful stimulus affects the nervous system's response to a pain arising from somewhere else in the body. Hippocrates himself said that 'the greater pain blunts the lesser', and until 1979 this astute observation, though frequently used in support of all kinds of counter-irritant remedies over the years, had not been thoroughly investigated.

Their subjects were rats that had been given a general anaesthetic to prevent them being consciously aware of any pain.

By careful dissection they placed micro-electrodes in those parts of the spinal cord that picked up both normal and painful sensations from one hind paw. Thus, stimulating that hind paw in what would have been a painful manner if the rat had not been anaesthetised increased the firing-rate of the nerve cells immediately under the electrodes.

They then stimulated various parts of the rat's body in a similar manner at the same time; these other parts of the body included the ears, muzzle, either foreleg, opposite hind paw and tail.

The experiment showed the remarkable fact that the normal response of the nerve cells of the hind paw was blocked immediately when a painful stimulus was delivered to any of the *other* regions of the animal's body at the same time. The experimenters coined the phrase 'diffuse noxious inhibitory control' (or DNIC) system to encompass this phenomenon. This means that there appears to be yet another method of pain relief that functions almost instantly, as opposed to the slower-acting endorphin system described in Chapter 12.

This diffuse noxious inhibitory control principle may well be a way of explaining the extraordinary variety of innately painful remedies offered in many parts of the world today for the actual relief of pain. Professor Pekka Pöntinen, who is pioneering the use of acupuncture in Finland, described a whole host of these:[5]

Cupping (where an empty vessel is applied to the skin and allowed to cool; this causes a vacuum which sucks the skin into the brim of the vessel, causing a large bruise) used in Africa, Arabia, China, Europe, Scandinavia (particularly Finland and Lapland) and India;

Blood-letting (where an incision is made into a vein to drain off blood) – Eastern Europe, Scandinavia and East Germany;

Leeches (an aquatic blood-sucking worm that can be applied to the skin) – Central and Eastern Europe;

Moxibustion (burning the skin) – China, Finland and Lapland;

Trepanning (making holes in the skull) – Central Africa where (according to Professor Ronald Melzack, a Canadian psychologist who has made many contributions to pain studies) patients with chronic headache kneel down in the village square and have the topmost layers of their skulls chipped away with a chisel; one treatment is usually sufficient;

Tattooing – Ethiopia (I have also seen crosses that had been tattooed on the calves of an Ethiopian patient who had pains in her knees and feet);

Scarring – parts of Africa.

In veterinary work

Firing – using heated irons, applied directly to the skin overlying tendons in horses to increase their mobility;

Tourniquets – ropes tied so tightly around the noses of Swedish cavalry horses (according to Dr Bengt Sjölund, a Swedish neurosurgeon who has made valuable contributions to the understanding of pain mechanisms) that minor surgery can be carried out on them.[6]

Sophisticated treatments

More sophisticated treatments are offered to patients in physiotherapy or rehabilitation departments. Most of these are uncomfortable, threatening or painful in themselves. They include in their number deep massage, traction (stretching the patient on apparatus that resembles the medieval rack), heat provided by hot packs, cold provided by crushed ice, liniments (ointments deliberately designed to irritate the skin), manipulation (where the joints are moved rapidly in a frightening and sometimes painful manner), painful exercises and injections of various kinds.

'Quaint' remedies

Even the wealthier countries in the world have their own quaint, 'natural' remedies of various kinds for painful conditions. In the countryside in Great Britain bee and nettle stings are still used for rheumatic pain. I remember a farmer's wife who had a painful neck; her husband came in while she was preparing a meal and plunged some stinging nettles down the back of her dress. This relieved her of her pain for six weeks, but she would not let him repeat the experiment.

The most famous British remedy is the hot-water bottle. Those afflicted by chronic pain creep down to the kitchen and fill this curious rubber bag with boiling water and apply it as closely as possible to the affected part; indeed, the hallmark of a British patient suffering chronic pain is a mottled pattern of brown marks developed in the skin as a result of repeated burns from hot-water bottles.

The fact that a patient in pain is prepared to tolerate a hot-water bottle that would normally be far too hot to be pressed against the skin is itself an interesting phenomenon.

A patient in pain often tolerates *more* pain than when he is well; in other words, contrary to general opinion, it appears that patients in pain have higher pain thresholds than when they are free of pain. This would also fit in well with the diffuse noxious inhibitory control system, as the pain a patient is already suffering would be expected to block the appreciation of pain from any other source.

Patients in pain hardly feel the needles

This is helpful to the acupuncturist, for patients in pain hardly feel the needles. In fact many patients in pain say, 'Doctor, I don't mind what you do, as long as you get rid of this pain.' They would never give another person such licence when well. Indeed, it is only when they start to improve that they begin to realise that the insertion of the needles may be slightly painful.

The noxious stimulus

Thus a new word is needed – *noxious*. This describes a stimulus that would normally be expected to be painful but which in actual fact does not hurt on all occasions.

A noxious stimulus is one that destroys cells within the body; this in turn releases their contents, which has the effect of stimulating special parts of the nervous system designed to respond to such an event. One can imagine this specialised part of the nervous system (the nociceptor or pain receptor system) acting as a burglar alarm, waiting to report any sign of damage to the body. Whether or not its messages ever reach consciousness depends on what else is happening at the time.

Even if the patient is not made aware consciously of a noxious stimulus, the 'ringing of the burglar alarm' (the increased firing rate within the nociceptor or pain receptor system) still has profound effects on many reflex activities within the nervous system, which control, for example, the circulation of blood and muscle tone.

The advantages of using acupuncture

If the only beneficial effect of acupuncture is occasioned by the noxious stimulus it produces, then in a sense the same approach is used by doctors who employ any of the methods that have just been described for the relief of pain; in fact those doctors who criticise acupuncture are already practising it, without realising this.

The advantage of acupuncture over some of the painful methods that have just been mentioned is that the noxious stimulus can be applied in a *precise* manner; the degree of pain elicited can be varied from nothing at all to any degree of intensity required for the relief of the patient's condition.

Also, the site of the needling can be chosen with great accuracy, as the needle itself is so fine.

Furthermore, various depths of insertion produce different effects: the skin itself is packed with elements of the nervous system that respond in a positive fashion to most forms of damage to cells nearby; similar networks of nerve fibres exist in the layers immediately below the skin, in the sensitive linings of muscles and bone, and also in the blood vessel walls supplying muscles.

Deciding where to insert the needle

We now suppose from the evidence given in this chapter that inserting a needle in the body at random (avoiding anatomically dangerous regions of course) would be a successful method of relieving pain in about 60 per cent of patients, provided the needle is inserted in the Chinese manner; this tends to be a deep insertion through skin and linings of muscle into the body of the muscles themselves. The needle is usually twirled and manipulated in such a way as to elicit a strange sensation called *techi* (pronounced 'derchee' and meaning 'obtaining the *chi*'). This may be experienced, according to Chinese sources,[7] in one or more of the following ways: *suan*, the 'sour' ache as found during heavy exercise; *ma* or numbness (this is the description given by the patient and is rarely accompanied by true numbness to pinprick, for example); *chang* or fullness; and *chung* or heaviness. On the whole these are unpleasant experiences, although those who have had several treatments look forward to them as they appreciate the relief they bring.

Most practitioners who advocate the classical approach to acupuncture therapy prefer to needle traditionally described points. In fact one method of deciding where to insert the needle is to read the 'prescriptions' handed down over many centuries; each 'prescription' contains a list of points that have been found useful in the treatment of any given condition.

Certain points recur again and again throughout these 'prescriptions'. These commonly used points are in fact tender in most people, whether they are ill or not. A classical and perhaps the most famous of these common points is *Hegu* (translated into English as the 'Joining of the Valleys'); this point lies in the hand (see Figure 21).[8] The reader may check

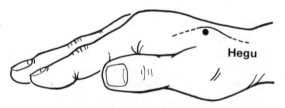

Figure 21   Hegu – *the Joining of the Valleys.*

for himself if deep pressure in the region of this point elicits tenderness.

The Chinese may have discovered two millennia ago that needling these particular points (which are usually tender in any case) is an effective method of invoking the diffuse noxious inhibitory control system that has just been described; this may explain why a migraine headache can be removed often in a few minutes by twirling a needle in *Hegu* in the hand.

Some practitioners like to learn the locations of these commonly used points from acupuncture charts.[9]

Exact location of points

Unfortunately it is impossible to look at a chart and be sure where these points lie in any given patient; for no two people are identically shaped.

The Chinese try to solve this difficulty by teaching the practitioner a special unit called a *cun* or *tsun* (a Chinese anatomical 'inch').

The length of this unit is based on the distance between various anatomical landmarks on the patient himself; the favourite one being the length of the middle bone in the middle finger (see Figure 22). A tall man would be expected to

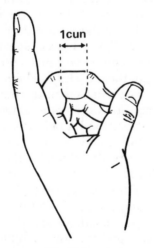

1cun

Figure 22   *The Chinese inch or* cun.

have long fingers, and thus his *cun* would be proportionally longer than that of a short man.[10]

Most acupuncture points are described as being so many *cun* or *fen* (a tenth of a *cun*) from such and such a landmark.

Yet nature has not provided human beings with such perfect proportions. This system of measurement takes no account of children, whose proportions are well known to be different from those of adults. I have observed the length of leg (from the joint space of the knee to the outer aspect of the ankle) to vary from adult patient to patient from thirteen to twenty-two *cun*, when the figure quoted in an authoritative manner (not permitting any variations) in most acupuncture books is sixteen;[11] while one book, *A Barefoot Doctor's Manual*,[12] quotes a figure of thirteen *cun* (again with no latitude) for the same length along the leg.

There is considerable room for improving the description of the exact locations of so-called acupuncture points, especially when one considers that they are meant to lie at various depths also measured in *cun* beneath the skin.

The nature of acupuncture points

Although some work has been carried out to show that acupuncture points are uniquely constituted regions within the body,[13] this is open to challenge; for we simply do not know where precisely we should start looking for them.

It may be safer, with the knowledge we have now, to assume that they are regions within such tissues as muscles, tendons and linings of the muscles and bones that are for some reason *more tender* on occasions than surrounding regions. No one knows why these areas should be so tender. Perhaps they receive a relatively poor blood supply (for they often lie in the extremities of the limbs, and as far as the muscles are concerned they are usually distributed either along their free borders, or at each end).

Nevertheless the Chinese appear to have spotted the remarkable fact that some regions of the body are tender in almost all healthy people; these are the ones that appear commonly in their 'prescriptions'. While those that are mentioned only in 'prescriptions' for certain diseases are usually tender only in patients who have those particular illnesses.

What is so fascinating is that tender points also appear in diseases which are not normally associated with pain; for instance many such points appear in muscles around the chest in asthmatic patients. These same regions are described in the particular Chinese 'prescriptions' for this disease.

Chinese physicians often treat both the particular and the common points; the former generally lie relatively close to the site of the symptoms, while the latter occur usually below the elbows and knees.

Tender points are acupuncture points

Tender regions within muscles have been the subject of special studies from the 1920s onwards both in Germany and America. Very little work has been carried out in this field in other countries with the possible exception of France. This work is almost entirely unknown in Great Britain. Dr David Simons, of the Department of Rehabilitation Medicine, University of California, has written a really excellent review of the work that had been carried out up to 1975.[14]

One of the most active researchers in this area of medicine is Dr Janet Travell, Emeritus Professor of Clinical Medicine, The George Washington University, Washington. She became interested in the possible role of tender muscles in maintaining chronic pain and other illnesses during the Second World War. She coined the expression 'trigger point'; by this she meant an area of muscle of which the patient was often unaware and which was somehow responsible for pain in another region of the body altogether. In other words, the patient might believe that he had pain in his hands, when the muscle responsible for this was in the forearm or even the neck. Likewise a trigger point occurring in a muscle in the buttock might 'shoot' pain as far away as the ankle; in this instance the ankle would be part of the 'referred zone of pain', according to Dr Travell.

She and a colleague, Dr Seymour Rinzler, published a set of thirty-two drawings showing the typical areas of pain felt by patients and the muscle regions they believed were responsible for them.[15] All but one of the tender muscle regions (or trigger points) in these drawings appear to correspond with the location of acupuncture points seen on the various Chinese charts. Furthermore in all but four of the drawings, the 'trigger points' and the referred zones of pain appear to be linked by the imaginary paths taken by the Chinese channels or meridians.

Dr Janet Travell did not need any special apparatus to support her findings; these tender regions in the muscles did not display themselves on X-rays, for example. All she required was a thorough understanding of anatomy to identify the affected muscles and her fingers to find them. She adopted the following procedure: she placed the patient in such a position that the muscle was gently stretched; she then 'snapped' its fibres briskly with her fingers. If the muscle was affected, the muscle would suddenly contract and often the patient would jump, complaining of severe pain in a region where he may not have been aware of it before.

Dr Travell used yet another stimulus – a very cold spray (ethyl chloride) applied to the skin. She found that the correct place to aim the freezing spray was not at the referred zone of pain (where the patient felt his pain was) but at the skin immediately overlying the trigger point (or region of tenderness within the muscle).

It is not impossible that the Chinese savants of long ago came to the same conclusions; although they explained them in quite a different manner and used acupuncture needles instead of an ethyl chloride spray as their form of noxious stimulus.

This idea was explored in 1977 by Professor Ronald Melzack, and Drs Dorothy Stillwell and Elizabeth Fox in the Department of Psychology, McGill University and the Department of Medicine, Royal Victoria Hospital, Montreal, Canada.[16] They ran into the problem that has already been described of wondering where precisely acupuncture points were meant to be located. However, when they compared drawings made by doctors who described 'trigger points' with the Chinese acupuncture charts they noted that all trigger points appeared to be in the same place as acupuncture points.

They then carried out a difficult exercise; they tried to compare the trigger points that would have been selected by doctors such as Janet Travell in the treatment of various conditions and the acupuncture points that were recommended in various 'prescriptions' for the same conditions. They discovered the remarkable high correlation of 75 per cent between the two sources.

In other words, Dr Travell and her colleagues (all of whom were unaware of the details of the Chinese studies) were coming to the same conclusions and treating the same regions of the body as the Chinese had been doing for centuries, albeit for very different reasons.

15
Infectious Diseases and Diseases of the Internal Organs Treated in China by Acupuncture

◆

The patient's response to needling has an effect not only on the painful spasms in his muscles but also on his circulation and other body functions through a part of the nervous system which is not generally under the patient's conscious control. This is called the *autonomic* nervous system; it controls sweating, the circulation and the presence of various hormones in the bloodstream. It also controls many of the functions of such organs as the heart and bowels.

Acupuncture and the autonomic nervous system
The noxious stimuli are known to have specific effects on the autonomic nervous system.[1]

Again it seems possible that the 'attention' of the autonomic nervous system can be 'diverted' by the noxious stimulus of the needle from continuing to give patients unpleasant symptoms; a simple example of this occurs when patients complain of a blocked nose. Needling the neck, face and tender points almost anywhere else in the body may relieve this within a few seconds.

We are entering a new phase in medicine where it may be demonstrated that the nervous system, far from protecting us from diseases, may be shown to actually make us worse than we need be. This attitude certainly prevails in the minds of doctors practising acupuncture in China; for they expect acupuncture to provide relief in many diseases where we in the West would not think this was possible. These diseases include such infectious diseases as malaria. At first the idea that acupuncture could be used to resolve an infectious disease appears laughable; however, some important work in the West has pointed in a similar direction.

Dr James Reilly and infectious diseases

Dr James Reilly conducted research for forty years from 1922 as the Director of the Central Laboratory of the Claude Bernard Hospital for Fevers in Paris.[2] He refused to be nominated for a Nobel prize as he wished to avoid any publicity for his work, which was at that time – and still is – revolutionary among medical circles.

He proposed that many events – including death itself – which occurred during an infectious disease were caused by the nervous system being directly irritated by the offending bacteria or their toxic products. He first thought of this whilst studying an obscure paper in a foreign medical journal in 1894, when he was only seven years old.

In his later work he noted that the poisons (endotoxins) produced by typhoid organisms could produce all the effects of typhoid when injected in minute doses into parts of the autonomic nervous system (in this case into the splanchnic nerves which supply the gut). Immediately following this injection the animal would produce the characteristic physical signs associated with typhoid. What was especially interesting was that if the animal had mild electrical stimulation of the same part of the nervous system prior to the injection, then these effects did not occur; while strong electrical stimulation made the animal die more rapidly. The Chinese themselves say that acupuncture should be conducted adequately but not too strongly.

Dr James Reilly's idea was that the nervous system is stimulated by the organisms to cause spasms of the blood vessels supplying various regions of the body, which in turn cause death. Anything that can dampen down or divert the nervous system from these effects would be beneficial to the patient.

He discovered that patients dying of blood poisoning would frequently recover if they were given a drug called Largactil (chlorpromazine), which has a marked sedative effect on the autonomic nervous system. Patients who were at the point of death would fall asleep with this drug and wake up greatly improved.

The treatment of malaria

It is conceivable, though not proven, that the needle effect of acupuncture may work in a similar way. In the treatment of malaria, for instance, in many hospitals in China needles are inserted a short time before the expected rigors (when the patient begins to shiver – thereby raising his body temperature). Following acupuncture the rigors fail to appear; at the same time the parasites are shown to disappear from the blood.

Perhaps the patient's rigors are a necessary trigger mechanism for the parasites to reproduce; we do not know. At least the rigors are not produced directly by the malarial parasites; rather, they are produced indirectly by the nervous system's reactions to the parasites.

The Chinese claim that the body's defence mechanism can be modified by acupuncture;[3, 4] a considerable amount of Western laboratory work is required to confirm or repudiate these ideas. If they are true, then perhaps we too might support the use of acupuncture in combating infectious diseases.

Acute appendicitis

Other remarkable work carried out in China suggests that acupuncture has an effect on acute appendicitis. The non-surgical treatment of this condition in China before the 1950s was starvation, bed rest, antibiotics (when available), pain-killers and sedation, together with an infusion of appropriate fluids into a vein to prevent dehydration.

For a brief period of time after the 1950s patients with appendicitis were given acupuncture at a point just below the knee and also in the abdomen; these patients were allowed to wander round the ward and eat at will and were not given antibiotics or intravenous fluids. Not only was their pain controlled but also the other physical signs of appendicitis, including changes in the white blood cell count, disappeared.

Dr John Lin Chung Zhi, a graduate of Peking First Medical College, who also studied in the Traditional Chinese Research Institute, described a report that has not been published in English:[5] 1,202 patients were admitted to hospital with all the physical signs of acute appendicitis. Six per cent had such complications as a burst appendix, appendix abscess or peritonitis (where the linings of the abdomen are infected); these patients were not treated with acupuncture therapy and were offered surgery.

The remainder received acupuncture therapy; only 6·7 per cent eventually required surgery as their appendices appeared to be perforating – while 1·1 per cent were also given antibiotics in addition to the acupuncture.

Meanwhile the condition of 92·3 per cent (1,109) patients was apparently resolved with acupuncture therapy alone. On average within 1–3 days after the treatment was begun, the temperature and pulse rate became normal; during the same period of time the pain and muscle tension in the abdomen were also relieved. In fact the temperature began to fall within 12 hours of treatment. Meanwhile the white cell count took 1–2 days to revert to normal. The average stay in hospital with these patients treated by acupuncture was less than 5 days.

Other studies showed that approximately 40 per cent of these patients returned with another episode of appendicitis within one and a half years. Therefore acupuncture is *not* the ideal method of treating acute appendicitis; however, as they could not afford Western-trained surgeons and all the materials required to sustain them, this was an achievement. Nowadays the Chinese will remove the appendix by surgery as we do in the West.

Experiments were also performed to see if placing a needle in the leg had any effect on the appendix. In both humans and animals acupuncture appeared to increase the normal movements in the appendix and altered its circulation so that it changed in colour from pale to pink.

The idea that needles placed in various parts of the body could affect the circulation governing the control of various internal organs is certainly not new in China – although it may be rather surprising to Western observers.

Diseases of internal organs

If one imagines a link between internal organs and the external muscles, as can be readily shown when an internal organ becomes inflamed and the abdominal muscles become tender – for example in appendicitis – then it is possible to consider a connection in reverse. The Chinese treat diseases of the stomach, pancreas, kidney, bladder and gall bladder with needles inserted into external muscles.

Should these diseases be treated by acupuncture in the West?

A great deal of work is required before acupuncture would ever be used in the first line of defence against these diseases in the West; fortunately Western methods have already been proved adequate for most of them.

Yet, if any of this is proven, acupuncture may offer us a new insight into the overall management of these illnesses. Certainly Chinese work presents a challenge to Western thinking, and does at least merit formal scientific investigation.

16
Should a Patient Receive Acupuncture At All?

◆

The acupuncture practitioner has to decide whether a patient should receive some more conventional form of treatment for his problem rather than acupuncture. In general, only a medically qualified person would have the breadth of experience as well as the training to make this decision.

Masking diseases
He must make sure that the patient has been adequately investigated to exclude in every reasonable way the presence of cancer, for example.

We now know that the pain associated with this disease can be relieved by acupuncture;[1] therefore masking symptoms of disease that are better treated by conventional Western methods is a very real hazard. There are two reasons for this: first, as acupuncture is carried out in a rather leisurely manner spanning several weeks, the patient may delay seeking the remedy he needs; second, the condition might become considerably worse before the patient seeks the treatment he actually needs.

Self-limiting illnesses
The next decision a practitioner must make is whether a patient will actually benefit from acupuncture. Some con-

ditions are self-limiting; for instance, certain painful conditions affecting the shoulders almost always get better within
a year.

In the list of diseases drawn up by the delegates to the World
Health Organisation Peking Symposium in June 1979 (see
Chapter 13), acupuncture was quoted as being a useful
remedy for the early stages of facial palsy (where a partial or
complete paralysis of the muscles of the face occurs); however, it is well known that the majority of patients who have
this condition recover without any treatment at all.

Patients who should not improve

Careful questioning will lead an experienced doctor into a
better understanding of his patient's condition, for there are
many patients who do not intend to get better whatever treatment they receive. This may seem surprising; but patients
often learn (quite unconsciously) to manipulate their families,
friends and doctors for the benefit of certain deeply seated
emotional needs – their illness forming a vital part of their
stratagems. These ideas have been excellently described in a
recent book by Professor Michael Bond, Department of
Psychological Medicine, University of Glasgow.[2]

Fortunately only a few patients are in this category, but a
doctor is usually fully aware of this possibility.

Assessment

At each successive treatment the practitioner should assess his
patient's progress. In other words, he should have various
yardsticks that help him to decide how severe the patient's
disabilities were before the treatment and what changes are
occurring as a result of the treatment. During the course of
treatment, if no further improvement is taking place, then
there is really no point in continuing with the acupuncture.

Today it is no use trying to use the Chinese traditional
methods of diagnosis as the only means of assessing a patient's
progress; the practitioner must at the same time have access to
the appropriate conventional Western medical investigations
(blood tests, X-rays and electrocardiograms) as well to see
what is happening. Thus the practitioner who relies solely on
traditional Chinese methods is in danger of subjecting his

patient to numerous treatments to 'balance' the pulse (see Chapter 4), when the medically qualified practitioner would have long ceased to treat the patient; the reverse might also occur.

Who may practise acupuncture in various countries

At this juncture it may be worth while stating that, in the United Kingdom at least, many medically unqualified practitioners of acupuncture call themselves 'doctor' or even 'professor' of acupuncture. Most countries maintain a medical register of qualified doctors; it is important for patients to check that a practitioner is in fact on the medical register before seeking his treatment.

In many countries, however, only medically registered practitioners may employ acupuncture; these include Austria, Finland, France, Norway and Switzerland. Doctors in France, for example, have been using acupuncture for 300 years. Many states in the USA allow only acupuncturists who are medically registered to practise. Germany does allow lay practitioners to work under statutory controls. In Russia, meanwhile, acupuncture is normally practised by neurologists. Sweden is the only country that does not allow its doctors to practise acupuncture except with special permission for research purposes; the Swedish authorities feel that state funds should not be diverted towards a subject which is so ill understood.

In Britain there is a strongly cherished notion that patients should feel free to seek help wherever they wish; thus anyone may buy a set of needles, start work forthwith and advertise himself as an acupuncture practitioner. However there is legislation in the United Kingdom restricting unqualified advice about prescribing glasses, attending birth, relieving cancer, carrying out dentistry and treating venereal diseases. Some county councils in the United Kingdom are beginning to introduce by-laws to make sure that lay practitioners are inspected regularly so that their standards of hygiene and methods of sterilising needles can be checked.

Pulse diagnosis

No one has succeeded in linking pulse diagnoses according to the traditional Chinese methods with modern Western diagnoses. Indeed, it would be a remarkable phenomenon if this were ever carried out; for practitioners who examine the pulse in the Chinese traditional manner are looking at disease in an entirely different way from those who judge a patient's illness by his X-rays, blood tests and physical signs. There is no reason why disease should not be viewed from several different angles at once; but the view of the disease from each perspective will be different.

As a result of the past two hundred years of systematic clinical observations in the West doctors are usually reasonably confident that a patient's illness which presents certain physical signs and test results will progress along a particular path unless treated in the appropriate way. Perforce this modern information is not available to those whose training is based on a philosophical system steeped in the culture of the China of two millennia ago.

Advice about drugs

The acupuncture practitioner must now decide how to advise a patient who is already receiving other forms of treatment, for most of the patients he sees have already tried numerous other remedies and are presently on some drug regimen or other. Chinese traditional medicine includes herbal remedies alongside acupuncture; yet some non-doctors often tell the patient to stop any drugs that he may be taking, on the grounds that these are necessarily dangerous.

A medically qualified practitioner would be aware of the pharmacological effects of the various drugs the patients are taking, and would usually be quite happy to practise acupuncture on a patient who is receiving drugs at the same time; when the patient's condition actually improves, then his drug regimen can be altered accordingly. This advice may well affect some patients' health adversely in a number of ways.

Some drugs, such as steroids, should never be stopped straight away. A wise patient should seek the attentions of a medically qualified practitioner with some knowledge of biochemistry and pharmacology; at least he does understand why a certain drug regimen has been recommended in the first place.

Miscarriages

There have been many comments in the acupuncture literature about the dangers of treating patients during pregnancy. It has been thought that miscarriages could be caused by needling; in other words, the nervous system responds to the needle by stimulating overactivity in the womb (uterus). On the whole, pregnancy precludes the use of acupuncture.

Dangers of acupuncture

Having satisfied himself that the patient's condition might be helped by acupuncture, and that he has been adequately investigated in a normal manner, the practitioner must then decide where to insert the needle and what dangers he may be subjecting his patient to in the process.

Before we consider what may appear to be a frightening list of dangers, it must be said that one of the strongest arguments in favour of the practice of acupuncture is its safety. Provided the practitioner has an understanding of the anatomy of the part he proposes to needle, and provided he takes reasonable care over the sterility of his needles, little can go wrong.

Under these circumstances in the treatment of back pain, for example, no patient will be made permanently worse by acupuncture; it would be difficult to say that of almost any other form of active treatment for this condition.

Nevertheless when these rules are not observed there are dangers – and these should be discussed openly.

The greatest danger of all to a patient is from an inadequate knowledge of anatomy on the part of the practitioner; for deaths have occurred from deep needling in the chest area, where the needle has been thrust through the ribcage into the lung and has been allowed to remain there for some period of time, causing the linings of the lung to be torn. The lung itself collapses as air is pumped into the space between it and the chest wall (a pneumothorax).

Other dangers may occur when blood vessels or internal organs are torn in a similar way. For example, cases have been reported of death caused by an acupuncture needle puncturing the heart.[3] Nerves may also be damaged by acupuncture needles.

A three-dimensional appreciation of anatomy for the practice of acupuncture is usually gained from the study of dissected cadavers at a medical school. A knowledge of anatomy is required to minimise the risks of inserting needles to a depth frequently recommended by Chinese sources of two or more proportional 'inches' (see Chapter 14, pages 145–6).

Serum hepatitis

Infections of various parts of the body may follow inadequate sterilisation of needles. One of the most alarming infections, serum hepatitis (causing a serious liver disease characterised by jaundice, when a virus has been introduced from the blood of one patient to that of another by an unsterile needle), is reported to have been caused by non-doctors in the United Kingdom in both 1975[4] and 1976.

In the 1976 episode a British Member of Parliament, Mr Sidney Tierney, described how a non-doctor, who incidentally called himself a 'doctor', used a mattress on the floor to examine his patients; he also had inadequate facilities to wash his hands. It was thought that his unsterile needles led to the development of serum hepatitis in thirty-five of his patients.[5]

This unhappy episode took place in Birmingham, and the relevant county council (the West Midlands) proposed a by-law in a Bill in an attempt to prevent this occurring again. They suggested that the rooms of practitioners who are not on the medical register should be inspected by the Medical Officer of Health and his team to make sure that only sterilised needles are used and that the practitioner is aware of the basic principles of hygiene.

These not unreasonable proposals were successfully opposed by a group of non-doctors before a Select Committee in the House of Commons.[6]

In the following year a similar by-law was proposed by the South Yorkshire County Council, and again this was opposed by the same group of non-doctors. On this occasion, a House of Lords Select Committee met to decide the issue.[7]

In the evidence presented before this committee there appeared to be considerable confusion in the non-doctors' minds about the technical requirements of the sterilisation of needles; for instance, they produced the erroneous idea that heating needles to a temperature less than boiling point was sufficient. However, they did say that in future all their members would use autoclaves (a thoroughly satisfactory way of sterilising needles – provided the machinery is used correctly).

The non-doctors also claimed that all candidates attending their courses already had sufficient instruction in the sterilisation of needles. However, inquiries made to the Chartered Society of Physiotherapists, some of whose members form an important group of the non-doctors practising acupuncture, indicated that no instruction is given to physiotherapists in the matter of sterilising needles in a typical school of physiotherapy in the United Kingdom – the West Middlesex School of Physiotherapy.

Despite the fact that it meant that a House of Commons recommendation should be overturned – a precedent not seen since 1908 – the House of Lords Select Committee decided to recommend that all non-doctors in South Yorkshire should abide by the County Council by-laws on this matter in the future.[8, 9]

Sterilising needles

Sterilising needles is not such a simple matter as it might seem at first sight:[10] the needles have to be cleaned of blood and tissues before being finally sterilised; this process in itself may infect the practitioner or other members of his staff. Great care must be taken in carrying out this exercise for a very small amount of infected blood can transmit serum hepatitis, which may cause much more severe damage to the liver than other forms of hepatitis.

Those doctors who wish to practise acupuncture ought to take advice from their local hospital departments of virology about up-to-date procedures on cleaning and sterilising needles.

Other possible infections

Other infections are possible. The Chinese advocate deep needling, often into joints. Orthopaedic surgeons would be horrified by the sight of a practitioner perhaps touching that part of the needle which is about to be inserted into the patient and the fact that the patient's skin is not cleaned with a suitable antiseptic preparation before a joint is entered.

It is the area occupied by the lining (or synovium) of the joint, which matters. In the case of the knee, for example, this is quite extensive. Anyone unaware of the anatomy of a particular joint may not realise that they have entered it. An infection of any kind in a joint is a far from trivial affair; its treatment may require a prolonged period in hospital and perhaps surgery.

Needling the skin and superficial areas of the body, however, usually does not require any skin preparation.

Frequency and number of treatments

There is some controversy about the frequency and number of treatments patients require. In China patients are often treated every other day for two weeks or so at a time; this is sometimes followed by a fortnight's rest to see what progress has been made; then another two week's treatment course is instituted if required. In this way a typical course of treatment may require sixteen treatments given over a six-week period.

In Britain doctors practising acupuncture often follow a different regimen; they take the view that long-term effects often follow each treatment. These can accumulate to the patient's benefit. Treatments are therefore spread further apart; a typical regimen would be seven treatments given at weekly or fortnightly intervals. The patient is told that if no noticeable effects have occurred after any of the first three treatments, then the acupuncture should be discontinued, as the patient is unlikely to benefit from an entire course of treatment.

The advantage of the British system is that fewer treatments are required. Indeed, with limited medical resources, it is not until the method is improved further and the treatments are reduced to one or two can acupuncture become available to large numbers of patients.

When patients are treated successfully a rather unusual phenomenon occurs with repeated treatments of the same sort: the first treatment may produce the most dramatic symptomatic relief, but it is usually short-lived, lasting but a few hours. The second treatment performed a week or so later produces relief that lasts for approximately twenty-four hours; while the third carried out after a similar interval of time causes relief that lasts forty-eight hours, and so on. On average, for arthritic conditions, for example, the seventh treatment produces a sustained relief lasting several months at least. In fact the aim of the treatment is to provide permanent relief.

Repeated placebo treatments generally have the opposite effects, every treatment producing benefits of shorter duration than the one before.

The time to stop acupuncture is when no further improvement is taking place. We will discuss the success rates of this form of treatment in more detail in the next chapter; unfortunately 30 per cent of patients who have osteoarthritic pain, for example, do not benefit from acupuncture therapy.

17
Which Patients Should Receive Acupuncture in the West?

◆

With these and many other thoughts the practitioner should calmly reflect whether or not acupuncture is appropriate for a particular patient.

A Western practitioner should confine his activities to suitable patients who have already failed to benefit from conventional medical methods; in other words, acupuncture should be used as part of the management of intractable, chronic conditions, preferably when the nervous system is intact.[1, 2]

The success rate with suitable conditions

One of the practitioner's first considerations is what success he is likely to have with this form of treatment. Table 8 shows the success rate of acupuncture practised by doctors in four non-Chinese countries: the United Kingdom, the USSR, France and the United States.

Table 8[3] shows an approximately 70 per cent success rate in all four countries; when patients are in pain, for example, the successful group implies a marked subjective relief of pain lasting for at least six months, following a course of approximately seven treatments given once a week or fortnight.

Table 8 *Results from medical acupuncturists in countries outside China*

Country	UK	USSR	France	USA
Total number of patients	1,000	10,700	1,200	1,800
Responses (%)				
Cure or great relief	43·9	32·7	68·0	40·0
Marked relief	29·0	37·1	17·7	35·0
Total	72·9	69·8	85·7	75·0
Mild relief	—	19·1	—	15·0
No effect	—	11·1	—	10·0

It is important to note that these were not formal, scientifically conducted trials; however, to achieve these excellent results the practitioners must have displayed their acumen in selecting suitable patients. These figures are greatly in excess of the 33 per cent success rate which is normal for patients who would react to suggestion alone.

These pilot studies do require confirmation by the clinical trials that have been launched in the United Kingdom and elsewhere. The results are not yet available.

Conditions where acupuncture is of use – arthritis and painful movements

Chronic painful conditions that often occur in the region of the neck, shoulder, elbow, wrist, fingers, low back, hip, knee, ankle, feet, etc., are treatable in the sense that the muscle spasms can be reduced, which alleviates pain and increases mobility.

In osteoarthritic conditions – where the adjacent bony surfaces are worn away over time – the needles are not going to alter the X-ray changes. One might well ask: How can acupuncture help?

Dr Janet Travell's work (described in Chapter 14) suggests that when pain arises in particular parts of muscles the referred pain frequently lies some distance away – usually in the region of the joints.

When a particular movement is carried out at a joint, certain muscles should contract and others relax.[4] However, if one or more muscles fail to relax, stiffness and eventually pain arises whenever a movement occurs that would stretch those muscles.[5] Strangely enough the pain is often felt by the patient to be in the joint and not in the affected muscle.

Indeed, it is possible that actual damage can occur in the joints if the muscles fail to function properly over a period of time.[6] The idea that damage to a joint is a sequel to muscle malfunction is not commonly accepted amongst doctors today; the usual thought is rather the reverse.

Nevertheless, this may explain why 90 per cent of patients complain of 'arthritic' pain long before any X-ray changes are demonstrated; the pain probably arises in the first place from muscles (which are not seen on X-rays).

Acupuncture may, in time, give us a valuable new look at the treatment of arthritis. Previously tender muscles relax following a successful treatment; much of the immobility, pain and sometimes the swelling over the joints disappears at the same time. Yet the internal damage within the joints is not remedied. Nevertheless the patient feels a great deal better.

Rheumatoid arthritis
Rheumatoid arthritis presents a different picture. Here part of the body's own defence mechanisms, the white blood cells, attack various structures throughout the body, including muscles, tendons and joint linings. During the active phase – which may last several months and is marked by hot, swollen, painful joints – acupuncture has little effect; however, acupuncture may be very effective in relieving pain during the relatively quiescent phase that follows, where the joints, though still swollen, are no longer so warm.

The underlying condition itself is not treated by acupuncture, and the relevant drug regimens should be continued as required. The damage that has been done to the joints cannot be improved by acupuncture, yet successful relief of pain is almost always accompanied by a reduction in the swelling over the joints – provided the disease is not in an active stage.

Headaches, migraines, etc.
Headaches of various kinds which come and go in episodes (for example sinusitis and migraine) may be treated. The

practitioner must exclude any infectious or even malignant condition which may cause these pains, and requires treatment in some other way.

Many patients with head pain have abnormally tender muscles in the neck region. Relaxing these with acupuncture relieves the headaches; again, Dr Travell suggests that the head pains are referred phenomena from the affected muscles in the neck or shoulders.

Medically trained acupuncturists usually quote migraine as one of the conditions in which treatment is most successful; they suggest that 80 per cent of their patients derive substantial, long-term relief.

This very high figure does require further investigation, particularly as the episodic nature of migraine makes any treatment difficult to assess. Nevertheless, the migraine patient might well consider acupuncture seriously as a method of relief.

When the nervous system has been damaged

Conditions where the nervous system has been damaged are much more difficult to treat. As has been described in the previous five chapters, acupuncture almost certainly works through the nervous system; when this is damaged acupuncture is less likely to be effective.

Nevertheless neuralgias where the skin is often painful to the slightest touch are often relieved by acupuncture; these may be caused by shingles (post-herpetic neuralgia) or by damage to the nerve supplying sensation to the face (trigeminal neuralgia). Here the success rate is much lower than that of osteoarthritis or migraine: 50 per cent of patients benefit – few are permanently cured.

Acupuncture will not have any effects in reversing diseases such as disseminated (or multiple) sclerosis, where the nervous system has been damaged. However, the psychological effects of acupuncture which have also been described (see Chapter 13) may help the patient tolerate his disabilities. Very occasionally patients appear to gain a remission immediately following acupuncture; it is always impossible to say whether this relief is coincidental or not.

Asthma and other allergic conditions
Allergic conditions such as asthma and eczema fall into the same category. Here the disease is not cured by acupuncture but may be substantially relieved, at least for short periods of time. However, at least half the patients suffering these conditions do not derive any benefit whatsoever.

Smoking and obesity
Many claims have been made, particularly by non-doctors, about resolving the habits of overeating and smoking. Again it is the psychological effects that may possibly be helpful; diets are usually issued or the patient lectured about the horrors of continued smoking. It is therefore difficult to know whether the remedy lies with the alleged treatment or the heeding of sensible advice.

Needles or other objects may be left in the ear for several weeks at a time in the belief that this may increase endorphin production (see Chapter 12). Despite the lack of evidence, endorphins are *thought* to be useful in reducing craving for cigarettes or food.

Some evidence, on the other hand (see page 115), has shown that obesity in animals is associated with an *over*-production of endorphins; if this is true, acupuncture would have the opposite of the intended effect on patients who are overweight.

Quite rightly, patients who already have problems with obesity may think that having a piece of metal implanted in their ear is an unnecessary hazard. Infection of the cartilage of the outer ear may readily follow such a procedure; the usual result of such infection is to cause a disfigurement aptly called a 'cauliflower' or 'boxer's' ear.

There is little evidence that acupuncture on its own can modify bad habits in a useful manner; in any case, treating the craving does not deal with the underlying psychological problems. Practitioners should address themselves to the extraordinarily complex reasons why one person puts on more weight than another or why one smoker lights up more cigarettes than another.

Conditions that do not respond well to acupuncture
As might be expected, more serious (or organic) diseases

where the cells of the body have undergone permanent changes are not helped by acupuncture. For example, poor results have been obtained with high blood pressure and such diseases as diabetes.

Here in fact lies a dilemma for practitioners of acupuncture. Those trained in Western medicine know very well that the insertion of a few needles is hardly going to improve damaged cells. Yet from the patient's point of view his symptoms (which are produced by the nervous system) may be dramatically altered by the acupuncture. Should the acupuncturist continue with his treatment, knowing full well that the underlying condition is not being resolved in this way?

This is another reason why acupuncture should be practised only by those who have had a medical training and have a special interest, where possible, in the conditions they are treating. Patients must be fully investigated to make quite certain there is no better method of removing the cause of their illness.

The holistic approach

Some may scoff at the contents of this chapter, as they say that Western medicine's obsession for separating patients into various disease categories is ultimately wrong; the whole body should be treated as one being, regardless of the aberrations of distinct parts that may lead to an artificially described picture of 'disease'.

The approach to the 'whole person' in medicine has been called 'holistic' (from the Greek for 'whole'); the word has become popular with the development of the science of holography (where a specially prepared photographic plate reveals a three-dimensional image when viewed with the aid of a laser light; if such a plate is broken into fragments, each part, however small, demonstrates a miniature version of the original image in its entirety).

We in the West have already built up our view of medicine in this way. We are now aware that each cell of the body contains the same genetic material as the rest; each fragment, in other words, already has (in our minds at least) an image of the whole. The interactions between cells have been studied by experimental work on the circulation, hormones and the nervous system. So we already have a grandstand view of the body and its intimately related parts, although we only have a small fraction of the answers to many of the questions we would like to pose.

The contributions that Chinese and Western medical studies may make to each other

The Chinese themselves have adopted most Western developments in medicine. Perhaps we in the West should look hard at Chinese medicine and learn something of use to ourselves – even though this process may pose many difficult questions about our own beliefs. We should not be put off such a study by the numerous misunderstandings of the subject. As Drs Lu Gwei-Djen and Joseph Needham so rightly say,[7] acupuncture has nothing to do with parapsychology, occult influences or 'psychic powers'; the subject does not deserve the praises of those who believe in such things.

As we have seen, the effects of acupuncture do not depend entirely on suggestion, nor on hypnotic phenomena, and do not contradict the findings of modern medicine.

Quite simply, acupuncture is a system of medical treatment which was developed in a very different civilisation from that of Europe and was already two thousand years old before the birth of modern medicine. For all its subtleties and valuable lessons for us in the West, the traditions of the subject are based on an understanding of nature which was not essentially dissimilar from our own ideas in the Middle Ages. It may never be possible to place any of these ancient concepts in a more modern setting.

Nevertheless, its actions can be re-explored by applying the methods of modern medicine: for instance, recent discoveries in the physiology and biochemistry of the nervous system allow us to begin to speculate again about some of acupuncture's mechanisms. The nervous system itself is so complex that it is almost certain that acupuncture's actions will never be understood in their entirety.

Yet we have a duty to try and unravel the mystery:

All phenomena have their causes. If one does not know these causes, although one may happen to be right (about the facts), it is as if one knew nothing, and in the end one will be bewildered. It was through this knowledge that the ancient kings, the famous men, and clever scholars, distinguished themselves from the mass of the people. The fact that water leaves the mountains and runs to the sea is not due to any dislike of the mountains and love for the sea, but is the effect of height as such.[8]

Thus wrote a Taoist philosopher in 239 BC, who begged the sages not to content themselves with the mere outward appearances of phenomena but to seek the reasons for them.

Yet those Western doctors who dare to venture into Chinese medicine must never lose sight of any of their original training. They should in fact use their scientific and clinical knowledge to distinguish, where possible, the truth from the dross of a subject so full of legendary lore.

References

$\blacklozenge$

Part One   Ancient Art *v.* Modern Medicine

CHAPTER I   SWING OF THE PENDULUM

1 Joshua S. Horn, *Away with all pests* (Hamlyn Publishing Group Ltd, Hamlyn House, Feltham, Middlesex, England, 1969), p. 45.
2 William Sewell, 'Early days of Western Medical Education in China', lecture given to the Europe China Association, International Summer School, Lady Margaret Hall, Oxford, during the series 'China, Medicine and the West', July 1979.
3 Ralph C. Croizier, *Traditional Medicine in Modern China*, Harvard East Asian Series, 34 (Harvard University Press, Cambridge, Massachusetts, 1968), p. 46 (also Wu Lien-te, 'Plague Fighter', Chaps 1–4.)
4 ibid., pp. 71–2 (and Ch'en Tu-hsiu, *Call to Youth*, tr. in Teng and Fairbank's *China's Response to the West*, p. 245.)
5 ibid., p. 73 (and *Selected Works of Lu Hsün*, Yang Hsien-i and Gladys Young (Peking, 1956) 1, 40–8).
6 ibid., p. 119 (and Ch'en Ts'un-jen, *Chin chin yu wei t'an* (Assorted conversational tidbits, Hong Kong, 1957) pp. 88–93).
7 ibid., pp. 191–2.
8 ibid., p. 192 (and Jan Cerny, 'Chinese Psychiatry', *International Journal of Psychiatry*, 1, 1965, pp. 229–38).
9 Joshua S. Horn, op. cit., p. 76 (and *The United Front in Cultural Work*, Selected Works, vol. III. Peking).
10 Ralph C. Croizier, op. cit., p. 154.
11 ibid., pp. 157–8.
12 ibid., pp. 162–74.
13 Joshua S. Horn, op. cit., p. 70.
14 John Lim, *The History and Development of Acupuncture* (The Seventies 1975, No. 5).
15 Ralph C. Croizier, op. cit., p. 202.

Part Two   Traditional Acupuncture

CHAPTER 2   TRADITIONAL ACUPUNCTURE

1 Yong Yap and Arthur Cotterell, *The Early Civilisation of China* (Book Club Associates, London, 1975) pp. 37–55.

2 Ilza Veith, *The Yellow Emperor's Classic of Internal Medicine* (University of California Press, 1972) p. 97.
3 ibid., p. 186.
4 ibid., p. 178.
5 Ilza Veith, *The Yellow Emperor's Classic of Internal Medicine* (University of California Press, 1972).
6 ibid., Preface, pp. xi–xv.
7 ibid., p. 213.
8 ibid., pp. 221–2.
9 Joseph Needham and Lu Gwei-Djen, Problems of Translation and Modernisation of Ancient Chinese Technical Terms, *Annals of Science*, vol. 32, 1975, pp. 491–502.
10 Ilza Veith, op. cit., p. 115.
11 ibid., pp. 126–7.
12 Joseph Needham, *Science and Civilization in China* (Cambridge University Press, 1975), vol. 2, p. 23.
13 Joseph Needham, *Science and Civilization in China* (Cambridge University Press, 1956 onwards), vols 1–6.
14 Joseph Needham and Lu Gwei-Djen, op. cit., p. 496.
15 Ilza Veith, op. cit., p. 184.

CHAPTER 3   MERIDIANS AND THE CAUSES OF DISEASE

1 Ilza Veith, *The Yellow Emperor's Classic of Internal Medicine* (University of California Press, 1972) p. 139.
2 ibid., p. 154.
3 Lu Gwei-Djen and Joseph Needham, *Celestial Lancets, a History and Rationale of Acupuncture and Moxa* (Cambridge University Press, 1980) pp. 15–18.
4 Felix Mann, *The Meridians of Acupuncture* (William Heinemann Medical Books Limited, 1972), pp. 21 and 164–73.
5 Felix Mann, *The Meridians of Acupuncture* (William Heinemann Medical Books Limited, 1972).
6 Nanking Academy of Chinese Medicine, *Zhongyixue Gailun (A Summary of Chinese Medicine)* (The People's Hygiene Publishing House, Peking, 1959).
7 Shanghai Academy of Chinese Medicine, *Zhenjiuxue Jiangyi (Lectures in Acupuncture and Moxibustion)* (Shanghai Scientific and Technical Publishing House, Shanghai, 1960).
8 Alexander Macdonald, previously unpublished.
9 Felix Mann, op. cit., pp. 143–6.
10 Alexander Macdonald, 'Developing Medical Acupuncture', *Acupuncture and Electro-Therapeutics Research International Journal*, vol. 4, 1979, pp. 43–9.
11 The Academy of Traditional Chinese Medicine, *An Outline of Chinese Acupuncture* (Foreign Languages Press, Peking, 1975), p. 133.
12 Ilza Veith, op. cit., pp. 157–8.
13 ibid., p. 165.
14 ibid., pp. 118–20.
15 Felix Mann, *Acupuncture the Ancient Chinese Art of Healing*, 2nd edn (William Heinemann Medical Books Ltd, 1972), pp. 176–80.
16 Ilza Veith, op. cit., p. 107.
17 ibid., p. 141.
18 ibid., p. 56.

CHAPTER 4 EXAMINING THE PULSE

1 Ilza Veith, *The Yellow Emperor's Classic of Internal Medicine* (University of California Press, 1972) pp. 172–3.
2 ibid., pp. 190–1.
3 ibid., pp. 172–3.
4 ibid., p. 163.
5 ibid., pp. 169–70.
6 Alan Klide and Shiu Kung, *Veterinary Acupuncture* (University of Pennsylvania Press, 1977), pp. 14–15.
7 Felix Mann, *Acupuncture the Chinese Art of Healing* 2nd edn (William Heinemann Medical Books Ltd, 1972), pp. 156–61.

CHAPTER 5 CATEGORIES OF DISEASE AND THE PLANNING OF THEIR TREATMENT

1 Jane Lee and C. Cheung, *Current Acupuncture Therapy* (Medical Book Publications, Hong Kong, 1978) pp. 163–8.
2 Ilza Veith, *The Yellow Emperor's Classic of Internal Medicine* (University of California Press, 1972), p. 221.
3 ibid., p. 221.
4 Alan Klide and Shiu Kung, *Veterinary Acupuncture* (University of Pennsylvania Press, 1977), p. 35.
5 Shanghai Acupuncture and Moxibustion Research Laboratory, *Handbook of Acupuncture and Moxibustion Therapy* (draft translation by Hans Ågren, 1974), pp. 254–5.

CHAPTER 6 THE FIVE LAWS OF ACUPUNCTURE

1 Joseph Needham, *Science and Civilization in China* (Cambridge University Press, 1975), vol. 2, pp. 232–44.
2 ibid., pp. 245–6.
3 ibid., p. 249.
4 ibid., p. 236.
5 Felix Mann, *Acupuncture the Ancient Chinese Art of Healing* (William Heinemann Medical Books Ltd, 1972), 2nd edn, pp. 78–9.
6 Joseph Needham, op. cit., p. 249.
7 ibid., p. 244.
8 Felix Mann, op. cit., pp. 77–107.
9 Ilza Veith, *The Yellow Emperor's Classic of Internal Medicine* (University of California Press, 1972), p. 111.

CHAPTER 7 THE ACUPUNCTURE POINTS

1 Ilza Veith, *The Yellow Emperor's Classic of Internal Medicine* (University of California Press, 1972), p. 220.
2 ibid., p. 107.

3 The Academy of Traditional Chinese Medicine, *An Outline of Chinese Acupuncture* (Foreign Languages Press, 1975) pp. 33–69.
4 Ilza Veith, op. cit., p. 118.
5 Li Su Huai, *Points: 2001 – A Comprehensive Textbook/Manual of 20th Century*, English edn translated by M. D. Broffman and Pei Sun (China Acupuncture and Moxibustion Supplies Co. Ltd, 1976).
6 The Academy of Traditional Chinese Medicine, op. cit., atlases attached to p. 299.
7 George Soulié de Morant, *L'Acuponcture Chinoise. La Tradition chinoise classifiée, précisée* (Librairie Maloine, Paris, 1972), Atlas, fig. 36.
8 Anton Jayasuriya and Felix Fernando, *Principles and Practice of Scientific Acupuncture* (Lake House Publishers, Colombo, 1978), pp. 192–6.

CHAPTER 8   INSTRUMENTS OF ACUPUNCTURE AND MOXIBUSTION

1 Alan Klide and Shiu Kung, *Veterinary Acupuncture* (University of Pennsylvania Press, 1977) p. 291.
2 K. Chimin Wong and Lienteh Wu, *History of Chinese Medicine* (Tientsin, 1932), p. 29.
3 Lu Gwei-Djen and Joseph Needham, *Celestial Lancets, a History and Rationale of Acupuncture and Moxa* (Cambridge University Press, 1980) p. 77.
4 George Soulié de Morant, *L'Acuponcture Chinoise*, Texte (Librairie Maloine, 1972) p. 201.
5 Jane Lee and C. Cheung, *Current Acupuncture Therapy* (Medical Book Publications, P.O. Box 4853, Hong Kong, 1978), p. 17.
6 ibid., p. 60.
7 Ilza Veith, *The Yellow Emperor's Classic of Internal Medicine* (University of California Press, 1972), p. 180.
8 ibid., p. 71, fig. 24.
9 ibid., p. 150.

CHAPTER 9   THE SUPERIOR PHYSICIAN IN ANCIENT CHINA

1 Ilza Veith, *The Yellow Emperor's Classic of Internal Medicine* (University of California Press, 1972), p. 220.
2 Theodore Burang, *The Tibetan Art of Healing* (Watkins, London, 1974) p. 67.
3 Lu Gwei-Djen and Joseph Needham, *Celestial Lancets, a History and Rationale of Acupuncture and Moxa* (Cambridge University Press, 1980), pp. 117–19.
4 Ralph Croizier, *Traditional Medicine in Modern China* (Harvard University Press, 1968), p. 114 and Yu Hsien, 'Hua T'o yuan-lai shih shen-hua (Hua T'o originally was a religious myth)', *Ta kung pao, i-hsüen cha k'an* (Ta kung pao, weekly medical supplement), no. 69 (25 December 1930); the original article appeared in *Ch'ing-hua Hsüeh-pao*, vol. 6, no. 1.

Part Three   Modern Acupuncture

1 Birger Kaada, Erik Hoel, Knut Leseth, Birger Nygaard-Østby, Johannes Setekliev and Jacob Stovner, 'Acupuncture analgesia in the People's Republic of China – with glimpses of other aspects of Chinese medicine', *Tidsskrift for den Norske Laegeforening*, vol. 94, 1974, pp. 417–42.

2 T. H. Huxley, *Collected Essays VIII, Biogenesis and Abiogenesis.*
3 ibid., *IV, The methods of Zadig.*
4 Russell Brain, 'Henry Head: The man and his ideas', *Brain*, vol. 84, 1961, pp. 561–9.

CHAPTER 10   THE BIRTH OF MODERN MEDICINE

1 G. E. R. Lloyd, Hippocratic Writings (*Pelican Classics*, 1978), pp. 93–4; translation of *Epidemics*, book 1, chapter 11.
2 Lu Gwei-Djen and Joseph Needham, *Celestial Lancets, a History and Rationale of Acupuncture and Moxa* (Cambridge University Press, 1980).
3 *Huang Ti Nei Ching, Ling Shu* (The Yellow Emperor's manual of Corporeal (medicine); the vital axis (or the mysteriously Effective Controllers)), probably first century BC with commentaries of Ma Shih (AD 1586) and Chang Chih-Tshung (AD 1672).
4 Lu Gwei-Djen and Joseph Needham, op. cit., p. 37. (Willen ten Rhijne, *Dissertatia de Arthridide*; Mantissa Schematica; de Acupuncture et Orationes tres: I. de Chymiae et Botaniae Antiquitate et Digatate, II. de Physionomia, III. de Monstris (1683) (London, The Hague and Leipzig).
5 Lu Gwei-Djen and Joseph Needham, ibid., p. 30.
6 Wyndham Lloyd, *A hundred years of Medicine* (Duckworth, 1968), pp. 62–5.
7 ibid., chapter 2, pp. 66–9.
8 ibid., p. 137.
9 Kim Bonghan, *On the Kyungrak (Ching-lo) System* (Foreign Languages publishing House, Pyongyang, 1964).
10 Lu Gwei-Djen and Joseph Needham, op. cit., p. 185; also H. Khoubesserian, 'Libres Propos', *Revue d'Acupuncture*, 3–4 (1965), p. 7 (a plea for the interpretation of acupuncture as a modern science, and for the abandonment of the classical theories of medieval Chinese medical scholasticism).

CHAPTER 11   SCIENTIFIC TRIALS OF ACUPUNCTURE

1 Ralph Croizier, *Traditional Medicine in Modern China Science, Nationalism and the Tensions of Cultural Change* (Harvard University Press, 1968), p. 237.
2 Walter Tkach, 'I have seen acupuncture work', *Today's Health*, July 1972, pp. 50–6.
3 John J. Bonica, 'Therapeutic Acupuncture in the People's Republic of China, implications for American Medicine, *Journal of the American Medical Association*, 228, 1974, pp. 1544–51.
4 W. Houston, 'Doctor Himself as Therapeutic Agent', *Annals of Internal Medicine*, 11, 1938, p. 1416.
5 Paul Lowinger and Shirlie Dobie, 'What makes the Placebo Work? A study of Placebo Response Rates, *Archives of General Psychiatry*, Chicago, 20 January 1969, pp. 84–8.
6 Henry Beecher, 'The Powerful Placebo', *Journal of the American Medical Association*, 24 December 1955, pp. 1602–6.
7 A. J. R. Macdonald, K. D. MacRae, B. R. Master, A. P. Rubin, 'Superficial acupuncture in the relief of chronic low back pain: a placebo controlled randomised trial', accepted for publication (1981) in *The Annals of the Royal College of Surgeons of England.*

8 Albert Gaw, Lennig W. Chang and Lein-Chun Shaw, 'Efficacy of acupuncture on osteoarthritic pain: a controlled double-blind study', *New England Journal of Medicine*, 21 August 1975, pp. 375–8.

9 National Institutes of Health, Bethesda, Maryland, 'Workshop on the Use of Acupuncture in the Rheumatic Diseases: Summary of Proceedings', *Arthritis and Rheumatism*, 17, 1974, pp. 939–43.

CHAPTER 12   ACUPUNCTURE ANALGESIA AND THE
ENDORPHIN SYSTEM

1 Peter Nathan, personal communication, National Hospital for Nervous Diseases, Queen Square, London, 1980.

2 Jon Levine, Newton Gordon, Howard Fields, 'The mechanism of placebo analgesia' (The *Lancet*, 23 September 1978) pp. 654–7.

3 John Lin Chung Zhi, 'The history of acupuncture', abstract, unpublished.

4 Bengt Sjölund, Lars Terenius and Margaritta Eriksson, 'Increased Cerebrospinal Fluid Levels of Endorphins after Electro-acupuncture', *Acta physiol. scand.*, 1977, 100, pp. 382–4.

5 B. Pomeranz, R. Cheng and P. Law, Research Note, 'Acupuncture Reduces Electrophysiological and Behavioral Responses to Noxious Stimuli: Pituitary is implicated', *Experimental Neurology*, 54, 1977, pp. 172–8.

6 Chang Hsiang-tung, 'Neurophysiological Basis of Acupuncture Analgesia', *Scientia Sinica* 21, 1978, pp. 829–46.

7 Chang Hsiang-tung, 'Acupuncture Analgesia To-day', *Chinese Medical Journal*, 92, 1979, pp. 7–16.

8 Peter Nathan, 'Acupuncture Analgesia', *Trends in Neurosciences*, July 1978, pp. 21–3.

9 Philip Rogers, Sheila White and Christopher Ottaway, 'Stimulation of the acupuncture points in relation to analgesia and therapy of clinical disorders in animals', *Veterinary Annual*, 17, 1977, pp. 258–79.

10 Tang Jian, Lian Xi-nan, Zhang Wan-qin, Han Jinsheng, 'Acupuncture Tolerance and Morphine Tolerance in rats', *National Symposia of Acupuncture and Moxibustion and Acupuncture Anaesthesia*, June 1979, Peking, pp. 491–2.

11 William Lowe, *Introduction to acupuncture anesthesia* (Medical Examination Publishing Company Inc, Flushing, N.Y., 1973), p. 82.

12 Lu Gwei-Djen and Joseph Needham, *Celestial Lancets, a History and Rationale of Acupuncture and Moxa* (Cambridge University Press, 1980) p. 227.

13 ibid., pp. 218–21.

14 Alexander Macdonald, 'Modern approaches to medical acupuncture', *MIMS Magazine*, November 1977, pp. 67–83; table taken from a lecture given by Dr Joseph Needham to the Medical Acupuncture Society, May 1977.

15 Felix Mann, 'Acupuncture analgesia. Report of 100 experiments', *British Journal of Anaesthesia*, 46, 1974, pp. 361–4.

16 Graham Earnshaw, 'China bursts acupuncture bubble', *Daily Telegraph*, London, 24 October 1980, p. 13.

17 Basil Finer, 'Mental Mechanisms in the Control of Pain', in *Pain and Society*, eds H. W. Kosterlitz and L. Y. Terenius, Dahlem Konferenzen, Life Sciences Report 17 (Verlag Chemie, Weinem, 1980), pp. 223–37.

18 J. Esdaile, *Mesmerism in India and its Practical Application in Surgery and Medicine* (London, 1846).

19 The Academy of Traditional Chinese Medicine, *An Outline of Chinese Acupuncture* (Foreign Languages Press, Peking, 1975), pp. 298–9.

20 A. Golstein and E. H. Hilgard, 'Failure of the opiate antagonist naloxone to modify hypnotic analgesia', *Proceedings of the National Academy of Sciences*, USA, 72, 1975, pp. 2041–3.

21 J. Barber and D. Mayer, 'Evaluation of the efficacy and neural mechanism of a hypnotic analgesia procedure in experimental and clinical dental pain', *Pain*, 4, 1977, pp. 41–8.

22 H. A. Nasrallah, T. Holley and D. S. Janowsky, 'Opiate antagonism fails to reverse hypnotic-induced analgesia', *The Lancet*, 2, 1979, p. 1355.

23 J. B. P. Stephenson, 'Reversal of hypnosis-induced analgesia by naloxone', *The Lancet*, 2, 1978, pp. 991–2.

24 Chang Chen-Yü, Chiang Chhing-Tshai, Chu Hsiu-Ling and Yang Lien-Fang, 'Peripheral Afferent Pathways for Acupuncture Analgesia', *Scientia Sinica* (Peking), 16, 1973, p. 210 (also reported by Lu Gwei-Djen and Joseph Needham, *Celestial Lancets*, Cambridge University Press, 1980, pp. 246–9).

CHAPTER 13   CONDITIONS THAT HAVE BEEN TREATED BY
             ACUPUNCTURE THERAPY

1 Bernard Millman, 'Acupuncture: Context and Critique', *Annual Review of Medicine*, 28, 1977, pp. 223–34.

2 Kumio Yamachita, lecture given to the Nordic Medical Acupuncture Association in Tampere, Finland, September 1980.

3 Mary Austin, *Acupuncture Therapy* (Turnstone Books, 1972), p. 2.

4 ibid., pp. 62, 187 and 230.

5 S. Yanagiya, *One-Needle Acupuncture* (The Acupuncture Association, London, England, 1956), pp. 44–5.

6 Editorial, 'When Acupuncture came to Britain', *British Medical Journal*, 22 December 1973, pp. 687–8.

7 Shanghai City Acupuncture and Moxibustion Research Laboratory, *Handbook of Acupuncture and Moxibustion Therapy* (Chinese Text, Commercial Press, Hong Kong, 1971; English translation and introduction, Hans Ågren, 1974).

8 *National Symposia of Acupuncture and Moxibustion and Anaesthesia* (Peking, 1979), pp. 1–2 and 53–7.

9 Academy of Traditional Chinese Medicine, *An Outline of Chinese Acupuncture* (Foreign Languages Press, Peking, 1975), pp. 247–9.

10 Margaret Patterson, *Addictions can be cured, the treatment of Drug Addiction by Neuro-electric stimulation* (Lion Publishing, 1975).

11 Vicky Clement-Jones, Lorraine McLoughlin, P. J. Lowry, G. M. Besser, Lesley Rees and H. L. Wen, 'Acupuncture in Heroin Addicts: Changes in met-Enkephalin and β-Endorphin in Blood and Cerebrospinal fluid', *The Lancet*, 22 August 1979, pp. 380–3.

12 Vicky Clement-Jones, Lorraine McLoughlin, Susan Tomlin, G. M. Besser, Lesley Rees and H. L. Wen, 'Increased β-Endorphin but not met-Enkephalin levels in human cerebrospinal fluid after acupuncture for recurrent pain, *The Lancet*, 1 November 1980, pp. 946–9.

13 R. H. Bannerman, 'Acupuncture: the WHO view', *World Health*, the magazine of the World Health Organisation, December 1979, pp. 24–9.

CHAPTER 14   THE NEEDLE EFFECT

1 Karel Lewit, 'The needle effect in the relief of Myofascial pain', *Pain*, 6, 1979, pp. 83–90.
2 The Academy of Traditional Chinese Medicine, *An Outline of Chinese Acupuncture* (Foreign Languages Press, Peking, 1975), p. 5.
3 Charles Godfrey and Peter Morgan, 'A Controlled Trial of the Theory of Acupuncture in Musculoskeletal Pain', *Journal of Rheumatology*, 5, 1978, pp. 121–4.
4 Daniel Le Bars, Anthony Dickenson and Jean-Marie Besson, 'Diffuse Noxious Inhibitory Controls (DNIC), part 1: Effects on Dorsal Horn Convergent Neurones in the Rat; part 2: Lack of effect on non-convergent neurones, Supraspinal Involvement and Theoretical Implications', *Pain*, 6, 1979, pp. 283–327.
5 Pekka Pöntinen, lecture given to the First Nordic Course on Acupuncture, Tampere, Finland, 1980.
6 Bengt Sjölund, personal communication, 1980.
7 Lu Gwei-Djen and Joseph Needham, *Celestial Lancets, a History and Rationale of Acupuncture and Moxa* (Cambridge University Press, 1980), pp. 192–3.
8 The Academy of Traditional Chinese Medicine, op. cit., fig. 39, p. 102.
9 ibid., two folded maps facing p. 298 (indicating the sites of frequently used points on the front and back of the body).
10 ibid., fig. 30, p. 94.
11 ibid., fig. 29, p. 92.
12 Revolutionary Health Committee of Hunan Province, *A Barefoot Doctor's Manual* (Routledge & Kegan Paul, 1977), p. 35.
13 Hou Zonglian, 'A study on the histologic structure of Acupuncture points and types of fibres conveying needling sensation', *Chinese Medical Journal*, 4 April 1979, pp. 223–32.
14 David Simons, 'Special Review, Muscle pain syndromes', part 1, *American Journal of Physical Medicine*, 54, 1975, pp. 289–311; part 2, *American Journal of Physical Medicine*, 55, 1976, pp. 15–42.
15 Janet Travell and Seymour Rinzler, 'The Myofascial Genesis of Pain', *Postgraduate Medicine*, 11, 1952, pp. 425–34.
16 Ronald Melzack, Dorothy Stillwell and Elizabeth Fox, 'Trigger Points and Acupuncture Points for Pain: Correlations and Implications', *Pain*, 3, 1977, pp. 3–23.

CHAPTER 15   INFECTIOUS DISEASES AND DISEASES OF THE
              INTERNAL ORGANS

1 Kiyomi Koizumi and Chandler Brooks, 'The Integration of Autonomic System Reactions: a Discussion of Autonomic Reflexes, their Control and their Association with Somatic Reactions', *Ergibnisse der physiol.*, vol. 67, 1972, pp. 1–68.
2 D. A. Buxton Hopkin and Robert Laplane, 'James Reilly and the Autonomic Nervous System. A Prophet unheeded?', *Annals of the Royal College of Surgeons of England*, 60, 1978, pp. 108–16.
3 The Institute of Acupuncture, Academy of Traditional Chinese Medicine, 'Clinical Research on Acupuncture Treatment of Malaria', *National Symposia of Acupuncture and Moxibustion and Acupuncture Anaesthesia*, Peking, 1979, pp. 43–4.

4 Chen Gongsung, Lu Zhenchu, Cai Gengqiu, Hu Aifang, Zhu liankui Ding yude, Nanjing Medical College, 'Clinical Observation on fifty-one cases of tertian malaria treated by ear-acupuncture therapy', ibid., p. 44.
5 John Lin Chung Zhi, personal communication, 1977.

CHAPTER 16   SHOULD A PATIENT RECEIVE ACUPUNCTURE AT ALL?

1 Felix Mann, 'Treatment of Intractable pain by acupuncture', *The Lancet*, 14 July 1973, pp. 57–60.
2 Michael Bond, *Pain, its nature, analysis and treatment* (Churchill Livingstone Medical Text, Longman Group, 1979), Chapter 11, pp. 93–108.
3 William Peacher, 'Adverse Reactions, Contraindications and Complications of Acupuncture and Moxibustion', *American Journal of Chinese Medicine*, 3, 1975, pp. 35–46.
4 'Epidemiology, News and Notes', *British Medical Journal* 2, 1976, p. 1144.
5 1976 Hansard, House of Commons, 16 December 1977, pp. 1174–185.
6 House of Commons, Minutes of Evidence taken before The Opposed Private Bill Committee on the West Midlands County Council Bill (H.L.), 13–14 March 1979.
7 House of Lords, Minutes of Evidence taken before The Committee on the South Yorkshire Bill, 12–14 December 1979.
8 Hansard, House of Lords, 31 January 1980, pp. 994–1016.
9 Hansard, House of Commons, 19 February 1980, pp. 322–44.
10 J. B. Walter and M. S. Israel, *General Pathology* (J. & A. Churchill, 1979) 5th edn, pp. 656–61.

CHAPTER 17   WHICH PATIENTS SHOULD RECEIVE ACUPUNCTURE IN THE WEST?

1 Felix Mann, *Scientific Aspects of Acupuncture* (William Heinemann Medical Books Ltd, 1977).
2 Chang Chen-Yu, Liu Jen-l, Chu Te-Hsing, Pai Yao-Hui and Chang Shu-Chien, 'Studies on the Spinal Ascending Pathway for the Effect of Acupuncture Analgesia in Rabbits', *Scientia Sinica*, Peking, 18, 1975, p. 651.
3 Alexander Macdonald, 'Modern Approaches to Medical Acupuncture', *MIMS Magazine*, November 1977, p. 78; figures taken from a lecture given by Dr Joseph Needham to the Medical Acupuncture Society in May 1977.
4 J. V. Basmajian, *Muscles Alive. Their Functions Revealed by Electromyography* (The Williams and Wilkins Company, 1978).
5 Alexander Macdonald, 'Abnormally Tender Muscle Regions and Associated Painful Movements', *Pain*, 8, 1980, pp. 187–205.
6 Louis Mercuri, Director of the MCV/VCU Temporomandibular Joint and Facial Pain Center, Department of Surgery, Medical College of Virginia, USA, personal communication, November 1980.
7 Lu Gwei-Djen and Joseph Needham, *Celestial Lancets, a History and Rationale of Acupuncture and Moxa* (Cambridge University Press, Cambridge 1980), p. 318.
8 Joseph Needham, *Science and Civilisation in China* (Cambridge University Press, Cambridge, 1975), vol. 2, p. 55.

Index

◆